PARTING THE FOG

The Personal Side of Fibromyalgia/Chronic Fatigue Syndrome

PARTING
THE
FOG

The Personal Side
of
Fibromyalgia/Chronic Fatigue Syndrome

Sue Jones

LaMont Publishing
Reading, Kansas

Permission to copy personal pages is granted; in fact encouraged.
Permission to copy poems must be secured through the publisher.

Cover art by Terri Adams, FMS/CFS sufferer
All poetry written by Sue Jones

You may email Sue Jones at
suemarie@osprey.net

published by
LaMont Publishing
P.O. Box 125A
Reading, KS 66868

Disclaimer: The author has made every attempt to be accurate in conveying information regarding FMS/CFS, but assumes no responsibility for errors, inaccuracies, omissions or any inconsistency herein. This book is not intended as a diagnostic tool. Please consult professionals for your personal health problems. Any slights of people or organizations are unintentional.

Library of Congress Control Number: 2001133002

First printing 2001 by Chester Press, Inc.   ISBN 0-9712175-0-5
Second printing 2002 by Chester Press, Inc.
Third printing 2004 by Chester Press, Inc.

This book is dedicated to all Fibromyalgia/Chronic Fatigue Syndrome sufferers who have gone before us. Few were given the assurance that they suffered from a legitimate illness. Many never even had the luxury of putting a name to their illness. Their silent suffering must have been frightening and lonely. I'm sure they would rejoice in knowing the silence is finally being broken. The contribution *Parting the Fog* makes toward that endeavor is in their memory.

Acknowledgments: First, I would like to thank my husband, Don, and our two kids, Curt and Kinsey, for putting up with me on a daily basis. No small task, I realize. Also, thanks to the rest of my family, who provided stimulating editorial opinion for this book, goofy though some of it may have been (you know who you are!).

Thank you to my friends Janice Briggs, Barbara Schlobohm and Chris Dieker for pinch-hitting as editors and proofreaders, and others who also helped in that regard.

A big thanks to Terri Adams for her enthusiasm and dedication to this book. Her willingness to share her artistic gift has been a real blessing to me.

Without my long distance friend, Judi Alexander, you would not be holding this book in your hands. She planted the seed in my mind and lent her support and encouragement from the book's inception.

El (Elaine Grapengater), thanks for being my favorite sister and another source of continued support as I wrote away. You should do a talking book!

Thank you to those on the Guai Group who helped me realize I was able to express not only my feelings, but theirs as well, through poetry. This was another spark that lit the fire under me to begin this book.

To all who were in some way a part of this book, I extend my heartfelt thanks. I know who you are and I will not forget your contribution.

To everyone who encouraged me, cheered me on, and expressed appreciation for my poetry - you were all instrumental in this book becoming a reality. I hope its words will help you as much as your words have helped me.

PREFACE

Each person suffering from FMS/CFS knows the frustration of being misunderstood. We know in our hearts that we deserve better. We did not ask for this confusing, debilitating illness, and would love nothing more than to be rid of it. But since it is chronic, and as of now there is no cure, we have no choice but to deal with it. This can be difficult, because FMS/CFS sufferers are hit with a double whammy. We must contend not only with ongoing symptoms, but ongoing suspicion regarding the legitimacy of those symptoms. These factors make it very easy to let misery prevail and hope fade.

There are two reasons for the title of this book. One is that this illness can make holding on to hope as difficult as parting fog. But the resistant fog surrounding not only the minds, but the lives of FMS/CFS sufferers need not stifle our vision. When we are able to embrace hope, the fog begins to part. This is the point at which we see not only what is, but also catch a glimpse of what can be.

Fix that parting of the fog in your mind. Cling to it. Allow yourself to dream of it becoming wider and wider, until the beauty of a full life, in living color, becomes your vision. By doing so, it is possible for it to become your reality as well. The first step is simply parting the fog and savoring the picture of newness that emerges.

I believe everyone with FMS/CFS is very special. I understand completely the challenges this illness is capable of imparting. This book attempts to speak to the reality of these challenges. I commend you for your strength of character in facing them. You each have a story to tell. Share that story with candor and confidence. Allow the words on these pages to be your soapbox. Use them as another way to part the fog. In this sense, the fog refers to the barrier to understanding this illness so aptly provokes. If this book helps part the fog for others in your life, let me know. I will dance a jig on your behalf (albeit a slow, crickety one!).

TABLE OF CONTENTS

Introduction

Chapter 1 Fibro What?   1
       Poem: Fibro Musings   5

Chapter 2 In the Beginning   9
       Poem: Disappointment 12

Chapter 3 What's Wrong With Me?   15
       Poems: A Visit to the Doctor 16
           A Patient's Lament 20

Chapter 4 The Monkeys on our Backs 25

Chapter 5 Playing in Pain   35
       Poem: Pain   38

Chapter 6 Cloak of Exhaustion   41
       Poem: Fatigue   44

Chapter 7 It's so Depressing   47
       Poems: Appearances 48
           Untitled   50

Chapter 8 Stumbling and Bumbling   53
       Poem: Lost It   56

Chapter 9 Oh, What a Night!   59
       Poem: A Night(mare) 61

Chapter 10 So Much Loss   65
       Poems: One Life   66
           A Bitter Loss 68

Chapter 11 Hanging In and Holding On 71
       Poems: Pill Taking Blues 72
           Never Say "All is Lost" 74

Chapter 12   The Ripple Effect   77
                 Poem: My Family   79

Chapter 13   Varied Reactions   83
                 Poem: A Friend   87

Chapter 14   The Faith Factor   91
                 Poems: The Robber   91
                          A Sufferer's Prayer   94

Chapter 15   One of the Guais   97
                 Poems: Guai World   99
                          One of the Guais   100

Chapter 16   The Power of Perspective   105
                 Poems: The Small Things   107
                          The Magic Wand   109

Chapter 17   Letting Hope Reign   113
                 Poem: Hope   114

INTRODUCTION

On the cover I mention both fibromyalgia and chronic fatigue syndrome. Many doctors who have studied these illnesses believe them to be one and the same. I also tend to believe this is true. For that reason and for the sake of simplicity, I will, in this book, refer to them both as FMS, as that was my diagnosis. When the two are separated, from the symptom lists I've read, I match chronic fatigue as closely as I do fibromyalgia, since extreme exhaustion is my worst symptom. I realize many CFS sufferers believe their syndrome to be separate from FMS, and I hope you will not be offended that I have included you in with us.

There are several excellent books on fibromyalgia syndrome (FMS) and/or chronic fatigue syndrome (CFS). They are very helpful in learning about these conditions and what we can do to help ourselves. We sufferers gobble up every word in our quest for wellness. But because they are quite detailed (as they should be) the people in our lives who don't really understand our illness probably won't make the effort to read them.

I wanted to write an account of FMS that sufferers could relate to and others could easily read and understand. To make this possible, I am keeping it simple and short enough to read in one or two sittings.

Brain fog is, of course, a frustrating reality of FMS. Forgetfulness, lack of concentration and confusion wouldn't normally be considered the best breeding ground for book writing. However, it's so important to me that a greater understanding of this illness be brought forth, I am stubbornly forging ahead and writing in the fog. Also, I believe my concept of FMS will be more true while I am still under its grip than it would be after the fog has cleared.

This then, is not a book about winning the battle with FMS. Alas, I have not reached the point of waving the proverbial victory flag myself. Rather, this is about the heart of the struggle. We are on a road we would never have chosen to travel. The journey is rough and fraught with unpleasant surprises. Although we sometimes feel very alone, we are all moving along this road together. We must keep hope as our motivator and wellness as our goal. My dream is that one day each of us will conquer FMS. At that point the struggles documented here will only serve as a memory of the anguish we left behind.

Because this is a personal look at FMS, I have given you an opportunity to make this book personal to you. If your hands are too sore to write or type, please enlist someone's help. I have given you this opportunity because we all experience symptoms somewhat differently. In addition, we all see this through different perspectives, personalities and circumstances. So glean what you can from my account, but make it YOUR story as well.

My purpose in writing this book is to inspire fellow FMS'ers through poetry, a splash of humor and an occasional moment of insight. However, my main goal is to bring understanding to family, friends, co-workers, neighbors; anyone who needs a greater sense of what the FMS experience is truly like. If your desire is to bring insight to some or all of the above, buy several copies and personalize them. THEN give them this book. Following are hints to make this easier. This will afford each of us a chance to open many people's eyes to our own individual experiences with FMS, as well as bringing about a better understanding of the illness as a whole. By doing so, we all win.

May this book be a blessing to you as we journey on together.

HINTS ON USING THE PERSONAL PAGE

FOR GIVING TO OTHERS: If you are only giving the book to one person, it may be possible to fill in the personal pages of this book, as well as your own. If this is too much, one option would be giving the book with the personal pages blank, and letting the recipient borrow your completed one. He or she would at least know your personal story that way. Or adhere to one of the following multiple book hints.

If you plan to give more than one book, fill in (or make one copy and type in) the personal pages & make copies to go with each book. You could attach each completed page to its blank counterpart. However, if you'd rather it didn't look like a cut and paste project, try this: make your own small booklet of completed, copied personal pages. This could be as simple or fancy as you care to make it. Even simpler, put copies of completed pages, or answers printed on a computer in an envelope marked

"My Personal Pages" to give along with the book. Alternatively, leave the pages blank, get together with the recipient(s) after they've read the book and talk over the personal pages with them. Finally, you could leave them blank and see if the people you give the book to are curious enough to ask you about your personal FMS experiences.

FOR KEEPING TRACK OF PROGRESS: Before filling in any pages, make several copies of each one. If you have a treatment plan, reevaluate completed pages after 6 months. Note any changes on your copied, blank pages and keep these in a folder. Do this every 6 months, and presto, you have an ongoing progress report. You could also keep a copy of your first completed pages in the folder. Label it "My Road to Recovery" or some such optimistic title.

Fibro What?

It has always been a struggle for me to explain FMS. I was diagnosed in 1997, so by now my family and friends have all listened to my feeble attempts to relay information about this illness and its effects. I am still, on occasion, faced with a situation where I feel it's necessary to tell someone I have fibromyalgia. Usually, this is regarding something I've been asked or expected to do, but feel ill equipped to handle because of pain and fatigue. While I would love to impart an accurate, understandable account of FMS, to my chagrin, I am disastrously inept in the area of oral communication skills. Nowhere is this more evident than when I feel compelled to reveal my FMS and I discover the person I'm talking to has never heard of it.

Due to the need for a short name to call people who don't have FMS, henceforth, I will dub them "Norms." This is short for "Normals" although a case could be made that no human being really fits that description. Anyway, this is a tragic sampling of my typical "FMS revealing" conversation with a "Norm."

ME: I have fibromyalgia.
NORM: Fibro what?

ME: Fibromyalgia. It's a condition that causes lots of pain
and fatigue and other symptoms.
NORM: Is it rare?
ME: No, it really isn't.
NORM: If it's not rare, I wonder why I've never heard of it.
ME: In this area, the medical community just doesn't get it.
Most of the doctors I've gone to don't accept it as legitimate.
NORM: (thinking to himself) *If doctors don't accept it, it
must not be real.* (saying) How is it treated then?
ME: Well, I pretty much treat myself. Even the few doctors
who do accept it find it difficult to treat. There are so many
symptoms to consider.
NORM: (thinking) *Hmmmm, she must be a hypochondriac.*
(saying) Oh, I see.
ME: Not enough doctors take FMS seriously and other people
don't really understand either. It can be quite devastating.
NORM: (thinking) *She needs to be under psychiatric care.*
(saying) I see how it could be.

As you can see, a combination of a verbal skill deficit, fibrofog (with its very own future chapter) and a complex illness,
render me a bumbling idiot in trying to convey an accurate picture of FMS. I've even seriously considered carrying a card
defining it to give to inquirers. But that poses two problems:
1. remembering to always carry the card with me
2. looking like even more of an idiot

Following is an example of the kind of FMS conversation
that would leave me feeling like a noble spokesperson:

ME: I have fibromyalgia
NORM: Fibro what?
ME: Fibromyalgia. It's an arthritis-related illness whose
main symptoms are widespread pain, stiff and aching muscles,
unrelenting fatigue and lack of restorative sleep. There are
also many other symptoms, as FMS affects every cell in the
body.
NORM: Is it rare?

ME: Not at all. Actually, I'm surprised you've never heard of it. I believe it won't be long until everyone is familiar with FMS.

NORM: Why is that?

ME: This is a very complicated illness. The medical community has been slow to accept it. However, many astute doctors and researchers studying FMS are making great strides in convincing the medical community at large that it is a true illness. Wider acceptance will lead to FMS becoming more well known.

NORM: How do you treat it?

ME: I eventually learned to gather information from books written by doctors with FMS knowledge. Then from this information, I basically chose my own treatment plan and found a doctor who was interested in FMS and would assist me in following the treatment. Even after I was diagnosed, some doctors just gave me a prescription for symptoms and told me FMS didn't exist. They were wrong. The American Medical Association, National Institutes of Health and the World Health Organization all confirm its existence.

NORM: That's interesting.

ME: If you are interested in learning more, you may borrow a book of mine or check out fibromyalgia on the Internet.

NORM: (ideally) Thanks, I'll do that. I do want to learn more.

Sufferers seem to be learning more, too. We are reading books, attending support groups and logging on to Internet sites. As a result, we are better informed. And knowledge equals power. Due to the efforts of pioneering doctors and our own persistence in becoming educated and passing that education on to others, we are on the verge of long-awaited legitimacy. We are experiencing a "coming of age" of sorts. While this is exciting and encouraging, it hasn't come easily. As a matter of fact, the word "easy" doesn't belong in the same room with FMS. It isn't easy to define, understand, treat, or live with.

I went to my stack of FMS books looking for a concise, universally held definition of this illness. What I found were nuances and even contradictions. There is little agreement as to its causes and effective treatments. This in no way diminishes the reality of FMS; rather, it suggests the complexity of its nature. It stands to reason then, that those of us dealing with this dread disease have a hard time explaining it.

From the books on FMS I have read there is general consensus on the following:

Between 75% to 85% of FMS patients are women.

3% to 10% of the population has FMS. (This is a difficult percentage to pinpoint, due to misdiagnoses, sufferers who remain undiagnosed and FMS co-existing with other diseases.)

FMS symptoms were first documented over 150 years ago, but the term fibromyalgia was coined less than 20 years ago.

Diagnosis is based on patient history, current symptoms, tender point examination, or more accurately (in some opinions), mapping of hard or abnormal areas on muscles, tendons or ligaments, and finally blood tests to rule out other diseases. No blood test stands alone to specifically identify FMS.

It takes sufferers an average of four or five years to receive the proper FMS diagnosis. (Hopefully, this outrageous statistic is improving.)

FMS is a legitimate, clinical syndrome/disease. It is very real. This bears repeating. We are not fabricating this illness. FMS is very real!

FMS is NOT the physical manifestation of depression or other mental illness.

There appears to be a genetic factor to FMS.

It's possible for young children to have FMS.

At this point there is no cure. However, after finding a treatment plan (there are no quick fixes), symptoms may be controlled or even eliminated.

Since there is much variance of thought regarding the causes and proper treatments of FMS, I will leave it to my gentle readers to discern this for themselves. I will discuss briefly the theory and treatment that I adhere to in a forthcoming chapter.

When I became ill, I found it mind-boggling that so many seemingly unrelated things could go wrong with my body. After being diagnosed with FMS, I was even more amazed that all of these things fell under one condition. FMS is a virtual kaleidoscope of symptoms. While they may be colorful, they are certainly NOT pretty.

From what I've read and experienced, the big, major players of FMS are: pain, fatigue, sleeplessness, brain fog and depression. While pain may be one person's worst symptom, fatigue may be the worst for another, etc. Included in the picture are a myriad of other symptoms associated with FMS which give it a dimension unique to each person. It's doubtful that any two of us experience the exact same symptoms. Nor are symptoms manifested in exactly the same way. This is not a textbook illness, but one with a very individual bodily response. Thus, each person has their own personal definition of FMS, some complete with expletives! For me, poetry says it best. The following is a poem I wrote about a year after being diagnosed.

FIBRO MUSINGS

Fibromyalgia – oh, what a pain.
But who can I find to hear me complain?
My body is aching, my brain's in a fog.
My muscles are weak and as stiff as a log.

Pain's shooting through me, its havoc to wreak.
Too often I find that I growl when I speak.
So many maladies are plaguing me.
Were there an escape door, I'd kill for the key.

My family's indignant, they think I'm a bore.
They can't understand that my whole body's sore.
A cloak of exhaustion is covering me.
But the mess in the kitchen is what others see.

Folks may think me lazy, unsociable, detached.
Or they may think a hinge in my brain has unlatched.
What others think is out of my hands.
But personally: I don't think even the cat understands!

"You're looking so well" is what my friends say.
"How CAN you be ill when you're looking this way?
With a positive attitude you'll feel just fine."
Could they be saying it's all in my mind?

Speaking of mind, what can I say!
Mine's NOT a good place for a brain to stay.
Although information goes there to reside,
When I try to retrieve it, it runs off to hide!

Speaking of hide, my keys do that well.
And when I walk in a room, why I'm there – I can't tell!
I miss birthdays, engagements – all to my shame.
Even missed my appointment with doc what's-his-name.

What can I compare to a fibro night?
My husband is snoring, my muscles are tight.
With eyes wide open, my thoughts explode
Into worst case scenario overload!

Old mister sandman is no help at all.
He's just out of earshot whenever I call.
At last sweet dreams swim in my head.
That is 'til my bladder nags me from bed.

Again wide awake, I now think to pray.
And I tell the Lord all about my day.
I give myself up to His love and His care.
And the hand I am dealt, I know I can bear.

I'll change what I can and accept the rest.
Each day I'll keep working to be at my best.
And when all's said and done, at the end of the day
I know even with fibro, I'll be O.K.

Chapter 1
Personal Page   Date Written 5-22

My main FMS symptoms, with #1 being the most severe, are:

1. Fatique
2. Pain - all the time
3. Sharp pain in joints
4. Brain fog
5. IBS

Other than #1, the symptom that has impacted my life the most is: Brain fog

because: I can't think straight anymore.
I don't recognize myself now.

How I usually describe FMS to others: Pain in joints
w/fatique.

What I would like to add to that description:
Pain all the time, can't sleep, can't think,
bowels all messed up.

My analogy of FMS:
feels like chemotherapy.

Rating my FMS on a scale of 1 to 10, at this point in time, I would rate it:

Mild   Moderate   Severe
1   2   3   4   5   6   (7)   8   9   10

Other thoughts or insights on this chapter:

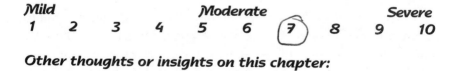
Wish people understood!

In the Beginning

It's fascinating to hear others tell how they believe their FMS began. Talk about diversity! Some have been ill with it all of their lives, while others were hit quite suddenly. It can strike at any age. FMS can creep into a life slowly and insidiously. It can remain an enigma for years. Many of us reach a point of desperation before managing to track this enemy down and call it by name.

Like many, in looking back to my childhood, I think maybe, just maybe, it began there. If it was there during my younger years, it seemed to have hung around unobtrusively. It gained a foothold my senior year of high school. This foothold gradually became stronger, until FMS made its grand entrance into my life four years ago.

My childhood did not stand out as an obvious prelude to FMS. I was raised on a farm, with an older brother and sister and both parents. We were all reasonably healthy. I was a fairly quiet, ordinary kid. Then again . . . . . .

I remember being excited to get all my school supplies ready for each new school year. And how I loved the smell of the new text books. Bounding off to school with new supplies and the heady smell of the books fueling my ambition, I would think: *this is going to be my year; I am eager to learn and I am going to study hard and be at the top of my class.* It never worked out

that way. Of course, it didn't help that there were a dispropor-
tionate number of "brains" in my class. Regardless, I was never
able to excel academically like I dreamed of doing. I always felt
different in that respect. Particularly daunting were math and
science. They kept me scratching my head and wondering how
anyone could actually get this stuff! Of course, it could be that I
was just at the end of the line when intelligence was passed out,
or perhaps I had a touch of ADD or some other unknown learning disability. Whatever it was, I felt my mind was blocked from
learning as others could. It just didn't feel like things in my
brain were connecting the way they should. I struggled mighti-
ly trying to concentrate, understand and remember. Through
most of my education my grades were fair ("fair" allows for
much needed leeway) but no matter how I worked at it, good
grades eluded me (except in music and english). Even later as a
young adult, I remember telling a friend I felt there was something wrong in my brain.

I realize we all have strengths and weaknesses and the
probability is high that my "brain problems," particularly my
deficiencies in math and science, were not related to FMS.
Certainly many people with FMS are highly intelligent and
have not experienced this kind of ongoing frustration with their
brains. Still, I can't dismiss the possibility of a connection
between the "blocked feeling" in my brain and the FMS symptom of brain fog. Often we display individual symptoms before
the full picture of FMS emerges. Since it is speculated that FMS
is always lurking in our systems, or at least the propensity is
always there in those who develop it, we can't rule out any early
symptoms as being unrelated (although I certainly don't believe
they ALL are). Nor can we confirm a relationship. All we can do
is look back at our previous experiences and if they are closely
related to any FMS symptoms, ponder the possibility of a connection.

Looking back at the active young girl I was is like looking at
a completely different person from who I am today. I could skip,
cartwheel, run, jump and play along with the best of 'em. Of
course, I may look a bit silly doing those things at my age! I was
agile and athletic, which would be a big boon at my age! I was

rarely sick. However, around the age of eight, I had my first stomach episode. It struck suddenly, like bullets hitting me in the stomach. I doubled over in pain. It stabbed at me mercilessly. I was compelled to lay on my side and draw my knees tight to my chest. The excruciating pain lasted a few hours; then was gone. This happened once every year or two, up through my teen years. What was it? I don't know. FMS related? Maybe. Intestinal problems are a definite part of this illness. While it made no sense at the time, thinking of it within the context of FMS and the problems it is capable of causing early on decreases its mysteriousness.

Since my brain experienced short circuit problems with schoolwork, I found my niche in extracurricular activities. I participated in all things musical. I was a baton twirler and a cheerleader. In junior high I brought home many ribbons and medals in track. We didn't have girls' athletics in high school until I was a senior. (That pretty well dates me, so you may as well know – I'm 46.)

I was excited to be on the school's first girls' basketball team my senior year. But around the time practice for the season started, I had to get my wisdom teeth extracted. I remember it being uncomfortable lying there with my mouth wide open for several hours. Also, I recall bleeding profusely into a can on the way home. Then I got dry sockets, which delayed the healing process. I never made it back to the basketball team. My gums did heal, but something was forever changed. I never mentioned it to anyone, as the change was subtle. But it was almost as if the blood that poured into the can on the car ride home contained part of my energy. I have never gotten it back.

I continued the rest of my activities that senior year, but everything required more effort. It was like every step I took was at a slight incline, until as the years went by, the incline gradually turned into a steep, rocky hill.

I have come to believe that people with FMS have always had it in their systems. It can lie dormant, or display mere hints of its presence for years. It usually hits with full force after a major stressor, either physical or emotional. So, to me it makes sense that a minor stressor (wisdom teeth extraction) would "wake up" my FMS. It moved from a position of relative obscurity to become a daily force to reckon with in the form of fatigue. Of course, I didn't know WHAT the cause was at the time. I just knew I was always tired.

In my mid-twenties, I remember times my husband and I had planned on going somewhere and I had to cancel due to intestinal problems. It wasn't the stabbing pain of earlier years, but pain none the less. For a time it came on nearly every evening. I also had painful menstrual periods, and came to discover I had endometriosis. Although I had laser surgery to correct it, the reprieve was short lived. It quickly came back, rendering me unable to bear children. It was during this discouraging time that I wrote the following poem:

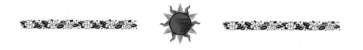

DISAPPOINTMENT

Disappointment fills my heart
But I won't let it conquer me.
I know if I only have patience
A better future I'll see.

There've been times before in life
I've thought my world would end.
But somehow I've always managed
To pick myself up again.

Life's so full of disappointments,
I don't think that I could bear it
If time didn't have the magical touch
To take the hurt and repair it.

Although things seem so hopeless
And life so rough right now,
I find my strength believing
That everything works out somehow.

At the age of 29 I had a complete hysterectomy. In comparing notes, many women with FMS have had hysterectomies at a young age. This seems more than coincidental, but there's still so much we don't know.

I've always considered myself an optimist, but in my twenties, I became prone to depression. I speculate this was due to the continued depletion of my energy level. By the time we adopted our first child when I was 29, I was in pain and exhausted. I had the hysterectomy when our son was only three months old, hoping that would help. It did relieve my pain, but the exhaustion remained. I chalked it up to being a new parent, gritted my teeth and carried on. We adopted a baby girl over three years later and I continued to concentrate all my efforts on raising our family. But the active lifestyle demanded of a mother of two young children took its toll. It became increasingly harder for me to make it through each day. What I was experiencing went beyond normal fatigue. It was time to find some answers. But those answers weren't simple, and they were a long time in coming.

Chapter 2
Personal Page   *Date Written* <u>5-22</u>

As a child I was: pretty healthy, but had constant stomach problems.

Now I am: Same way, but not healthy any more.

Looking back, I see these hints of FMS in my childhood: (some of you will answer "none")

Stomach problems
Unexplained rashes
Not as much energy as other kids

I first became concerned about my health when:

I was <u>tired</u> all the time.

This (or these) stressor(s) triggered my FMS:

Hepatitis C & Chemo. / Sarcoidosis
Divorce   / Too many stressors

My first symptoms of FMS began this many years ago:

1-5   (6-10)   11-20   21-30   31-40   41-50   over 50

I've had "full blown" FMS this many years:

1-5   6-10   11-20   21-30   31-40   (41-50)   over 50

Other thoughts or insights on this chapter:

None.

What's Wrong With Me?

From my mid-twenties on, I would periodically make trips to various doctors, hoping they could tell me why I was so fatigued. They had no answers. When I was around thirty, I asked for a blood test to see if it would indicate hypothyroidism. It came back negative. In my late thirties and early forties, more symptoms emerged. I was not only exhausted, I felt faint. My back hurt. I had chronic sinus infections and couldn't breath at night. I was becoming very constipated. I felt weaker and weaker and didn't know where to turn for help. My trips to the doctor became more frequent. Or should I say, my trips to the doctors. I went to many trying to find answers, while getting nowhere.

Mine is not an isolated scenario. Many with FMS search for years and like myself, are left confused and desperate for much longer than should ever be necessary.

Since doctor visits become such a vital part of our lives, some of you FMS'ers may relate to this slightly, and only slightly, embellished poem. I wrote it after an interminably long wait at a doctor's office:

A VISIT TO THE DOCTOR

I'm gonna be late to the doctor.
Hurry up, let's go.
I don't want to make him wait.
His time is valuable, you know.

Here we are, just in time.
I'll tell the receptionist I'm here.
She points me to a chair and says,
"Wait here a bit, my dear."

I leaf through all the magazines.
They're old as original sin.
But that's OK, 'cause I'm just sure
That soon they'll call me in.

My third time through the magazines
They finally call my name,
And march me to a little room.
"He'll be in soon," they claim.

Slowly time passes by
In the room with nothing to do.
My watch says almost four o'clock,
My appointment was at two.

When I've counted the squares on the ceiling,
Boredom turns into fright.
They've all gone home and forgotten me,
I'm stuck here the rest of the night!

Just when I'm about to scream,
"Someone get me out of here!"
Lo and behold, through the door
The doctor does appear.

By then I'm just a nervous wreck,
Practically delirious.
He says, "You don't look good at all,
It must be something serious."

"We'll have to run extensive tests.
Come back in a week or so.
You may dress, but hurry please,
I close at five, you know."

Honestly, I believe being a doctor is a very noble profession. Doctors help countless people every day. But, owing for exceptions, most people with FMS have not had particularly good experiences with doctors, myself included. Because the medical profession couldn't figure out what was wrong with me, they couldn't really help me. And I was in critical need of help. Unfortunately, I wasn't taken seriously. I had the strong sense they felt I was a hypochondriac.

Sometimes I was so weak and shaky and sick I was rushed to the doctor, only to be told to go home and rest! My constipation became so bad I ended up in the ER with an impacted bowel. That was the most torturous day of my life. The pain and anguish were indescribable. After that, I bought a book on hypothyroidism, as I'd heard it could cause constipation. The other symptoms fit as well. I took the book to my doctor and demanded a TSH test. This is a more accurate test than the one I'd had several years before. Not surprisingly, I had a severe case of hypothyroidism. Why none of my doctors had thought to run this test on me when my symptoms were so severe continues to baffle me. I lost a great deal of faith in the medical profession at that point.

The good news was I was told there was medication that would make me feel "like a whole new person." I had no reason to doubt that claim. I was thrilled that I could be essentially cured. I rushed to the pharmacy and started taking the Synthroid right away. If ever the placebo affect would have worked on me, it would have been then. I knew I had my answer at last. Best of all, they said the change would be immediate. A lottery winner could not have been more excited than I was in taking that first pill. But nothing happened. So I took them a few more days, thinking I was just slow to respond. Nothing. I still felt awful. So I went back to the doctor again, only to find my TSH level had been corrected by the Synthroid. I was beside myself. Why was I not feeling better? Was I crazy? What was going on? Again, no answers.

At this time, in my despair, I wrote the following on a piece of paper that I've kept, dated 3-10-97. I've a strong hunch, nearly every person with FMS, at some point before knowing, could have written something very similar.

> *My mind is constantly pondering what could be wrong with me. Why am I not progressing to the logical outcome of my thyroid treatment? Will there be an end to my suffering, or am I a freakish case that doctors will simply shake their heads at in dismay? Am I dying? Sometimes I feel I'm walking through my days never knowing if there will be a serpent under my next step.*
>
> *Everything is hard: Fixing dinner, shopping, doing laundry, dishes, keeping the house half-way picked up and clean. Some things are nearly impossible: staying awake all day, having fun, being a good mother and wife. I'm trying so hard to stay in the game, although my body keeps screaming FORFEIT, FORFEIT! All the people I love are here and I want to stay with them. They need me. So I will continue to try, always try. My future is a mystery. God alone knows what it holds. I am so grateful to know it's in His hands, and will forever be.*

After several more trips to my doctor of the moment, he sent me to an endocrinologist, specializing in endocrine glands, including the thyroid. He ran tests, asked about my symptoms, listened to my story and was immediately able to tell me what was wrong. I had fibromyalgia. Never had I heard the word before.

It was such a relief to put a name to my suffering and know I wasn't crazy after all. He gave me some basic information and told me to learn all I could about FMS. I am forever grateful to this doctor for moving out of his specialty and diagnosing me with an illness that no other doctor had ever even mentioned to me. His name is Dr. Wynne and he certainly is a winner in my book.

Later I went to a rheumatologist who confirmed my diagnosis, but he didn't have much else to offer. As I researched FMS/CFS, I was amazed. I found myself on every page I read. I finally felt validated as I learned all that was happening to me wasn't just in my head.

I learned that my "full blown" FMS was likely triggered by the trauma of my day in the ER with the impacted bowel (a major stressor). I find it disconcerting to know this incident, which triggered my major FMS, most likely never would have happened had I been diagnosed with hypothyroidism sooner.

Putting a name to the misery I still felt after my hypothyroidism had been treated was comforting. However, the term fibromyalgia didn't translate as an ah-ha moment for my hometown doctors. Actually, reporting my diagnosis to them proved just another roadblock. They didn't even accept FMS as a legitimate illness and certainly didn't know how to treat it (or from their view, me). They gave me scripts for pain, depression, sleep and various other ailments, then sent me on my way. I take none of these prescriptions now, as I actually got worse on all that medication.

My experiences with disbelieving doctors prompted the following poem:

A PATIENT'S LAMENT

I'm here at the doctor's once again
And I can't say I'm taken seriously.
I'm greeted with, "It's you again,"
While the doc's eyes roll up mysteriously.

"Doc, I'm so tired and ache everywhere,
For months I've not been feeling well.
Can't sleep, head hurts, in pain, I'm a wreck.
What could be wrong with me, doc, can you tell?"

He hears my concerns with a casual air,
Then says to the nurse as he turns his back,
"She's here all the time with the same complaints,
Your typical hypochondriac."

His eyes accusing, he looks back at me
And asks, "Is there tension at home?
Stress could be the culprit, so I'll recommend,
Relax, take a bath in some foam."

Not long 'till I'm back, no improvement to note.
Tension hangs thick in the air.
He thinks I'm one note short of a tune.
And I think he just doesn't care.

He scratches his chin and contemplates
How he can get rid of me once and for all.
Then writes an Rx, says, "It could be depression,
Give it some time before you call."

Information on fibro then crosses my path.
Each symptom fits like a glove on a hand.
So I march to the doctor, with me now accusing.
"What about this!" I demand.

"You've been told you have fibromyalgia," he says,
"There's no such thing, it's a wastebasket term."
While I agree that it's a "trashy" disease,
His take on it makes me squirm.

He proceeds to explain that reliable tests
Rule out all legitimate causes.
"Symptoms then left with no proof of disease
Are called that," he says, then he pauses.

"I just can't help you, I'm sorry to say.
Where there's no disease, there's no cure.
You'll have to take charge of your health yourself."
On that we agree, that's for sure.

So, here I am tired and aching and worn,
Taking charge of what my doc is not.
Certainly not a good spot to be in,
But I'm giving it my best shot.

So doctors take note as I conquer this challenge.
This is a war I will win.
If I can convince you this illness is real,
There's no better way to begin.

I don't go to doctors for my FMS much anymore. I do have a
doctor now who recognizes FMS and writes me a script for the
treatment I've chosen. For that I am grateful.

Nearly every person with FMS has "horror stories" of experiences with doctors. We have been told we are: depressed, just
fine, exaggerating, stressed, responsible for our symptoms – that
it's all in our heads – you name it. Some of us go many years
being called everything but what we are: FMS sufferers.

Before we are diagnosed, it's not uncommon for us to spend
hundreds, if not thousands, of dollars in our search for an

answer. Add to this the precious time taken away from home or work waiting in doctor's office after doctor's office and still getting nowhere.

This carnage continues until, at last, we find that one doctor who validates us by finally giving us an answer to the question "What's wrong with me?" Ideally, they then assist us in finding a road to wellness. God bless that doctor. May his/her kind greatly increase in number.

Chapter 3
Personal Page   *Date Written* _____

It took _15_ **years from the start of symptoms, for my FMS to be diagnosed.**

I saw approximately _5_ **doctors before being correctly diagnosed.**

I was diagnosed with FMS/CFS _1_ **years ago.**

Most doctors I went to with my complaints told me:
You're just depressed.
Exercise!
Deal with it.

The doctor who diagnosed me is: name: ~~Dr. Petsome~~
                                   title: Dr. Max

My current doctor's belief in FMS is: that it's not
                                          all in my head.

I'm on this many medications for FMS symptoms _3_ .
          Antidepressants, Celebrex, ?

I wish my doctor knew: how much it hurts, how
                           depressing it is, how the
              thought of exercising makes me hurt.

Other thoughts or insights on this chapter:

The Monkeys on
Our Backs

W e FMS'ers have all kinds of monkeys hanging on our backs. There are, of course, the main monkeys (symptoms) to which I've already alluded. As you read on, you will see that they have all earned the dubious honor of their own chapter. But since this chapter takes a more inclusive look at FMS symptoms, I will mention them here also. The big bads of FMS are: widespread pain, exhaustion, brain fog, depression and lack of restorative sleep. You would think these would be enough to make us sufficiently miserable. And indeed, they would be. But that's not all folks!

All of our monkeys have certain stressors which rile them up and cause them to kick and bite with added fervor. Among them: weather changes, cold drafts and rain. Like arthritis, FMS can be an accurate predictor of changing weather. We could give our morning weatherperson some stiff (pun) competition! Daily emotional or mental stress can also aggravate FMS symptoms. It can be difficult to reduce stress when FMS itself is a stressful illness in every imaginable way. Too much exercise, repetitive motion and sitting or standing in one position for prolonged periods of time can all wreak havoc on us as well. I personally have a "stand limit" of about thirty minutes, before the pain monkey starts kicking me hard in my lower back.

People often have FMS along with other conditions or
diseases; notably, auto-immune disorders such as rheumatoid
arthritis or lupus. Hypoglycemia often goes hand in hand with
FMS. Actually, FMS can be present with any illness or condition
and symptoms can overlap.

There seems no end to FMS's manifestations. Its monkeys
are many and relentless. We all dread flares, which are times
when our symptoms get considerably worse. Flares can be
brought on by the stressors mentioned above, or they can
appear with no apparent provocation. We do need to be careful
to not always attribute everything to FMS. There are many
unrelated reasons for the appearance of individual symptoms
that may fit the FMS profile.

Since there are so many problems related to FMS, I'm sure
I will inadvertently leave out some of them. I apologize to anyone who suffers greatly from a symptom left unmentioned here.

The large array of FMS monkeys can each cause major difficulties to those facing them. The following quotes are posts
from an Internet support group which describe some symptoms.
They may relay a better overall picture of what we are dealing
with. Some of them were posted a few years ago and the symptom mentioned has since been helped or eliminated with treatment (see Chapter 15).

In my estimation, the runner up to the major league symptoms is (drum roll) irritable bowel syndrome or IBS. This is a
huge dilemma for some. Included in this lovely package can be:
constipation and/or diarrhea, gas or bloating, severe intestinal
pain, and hyperacidity. Discomfort, thy name is IBS. Its nature
can keep you close to home. Its suddenness can cause public
embarrassment and its misery can know no bounds. An FMS
friend of mine is afflicted with the more rare symptom of nausea. Here is her description:

> *"Nausea was my first symptom. It started after gall
> bladder surgery, and never went away. The GI doctors ran
> lots of tests and couldn't find anything wrong. But I still
> got sick. There is no trigger, food or otherwise. The nausea
> just comes like a wave and knocks me over. Most times I'm*

sick for several hours to several days. I have tried every available medication and nothing works for me. My calendar is up in the air. I have had to cancel many plans due to bouts of nausea."   *Carol*

Vulvodynia is a big word for the more personal female symptoms of FMS. These may include itching, pain or burning of the vaginal area, painful menstrual periods, painful intercourse, various intense cramping, overactive bladder and other bladder disorders or infections.

Our muscles not only cause pain and general aching, they can do a number on us in other ways as well. Nearly every person with FMS experiences muscle stiffness, particularly in the morning or after being in one position for a time. It can affect us in ways a "Norm" would never even imagine.

"How about the mornings? With all the stiffness I can't get to the bathroom soon enough."   *Janie*

"I have the HORRIBLE morning stiffness thing (today being exceptionally worse, and I'm trying to think if I finished that marathon that I was in yesterday (LOL!). I also have evening stiffness as well. I know that if I sit on the couch for extended periods of time, I have to get up "in stages" to go to the bathroom. Like: sit up straight, pause, move to the edge of the couch, pause, stand up but don't straighten up, pause, straighten up, pause, attempt to walk."
                              Heather H.

(By the way, LOL stands for Laughing out Loud.)

Muscle weakness is also a frustrating fact of FMS. This becomes most obvious while trying to use our hands and arms.

"I love to read but have a problem holding up books. I am a school teacher and writing is part of my daily life. At the end of the day, I find it difficult to write. Thank God for computers, so I no longer have to write up all my planning. Opening jars is easy – I just call out to my husband!"   Wendy

We may experience excruciating leg cramps. These are mostly at night, where we have the advantage of probably not being asleep anyway! Foot cramps and pains may occur day or night. Here's another way our muscles may get our attention:

"Fasciculations: spontaneous irregular discharge of motor neurons that cause irregular twitchings or contractions of individual muscle fiber or muscle bundles. I feel these mostly as irregular twitching and sometimes as a feeling of muscle cramping. They are not like a complete cramp. I have had these constantly for the last 4-5 months and they get more frequent and uncomfortable with increased activity."   Donna B.

Chest pain is nothing to fool around with. If you experience this, it is wise to get yourself to a doctor. However, this can be FMS related. I have had two scary incidents in which I felt I might have been having a heart attack. This is not unusual in FMS.

"There are muscles in-between each rib called intercostal muscles, and they can spasm so badly from FMS that they feel like a heart attack. I have actually been hospitalized two times with chest pain, arm /shoulder pain and extreme shortness of breath. All of which indicated a heart attack. The ER kept me overnight in spite of normal cardiac enzymes."   Bonnie

If eyes are the mirror to the soul, then we are in trouble! We may experience irritated, burning eyes or burning tears. Dryness is a big problem.

> *"I have extremely dry eyes and also get the gunk in the corners of my eyes. I have to clean out the corners once or twice a day. My eyes are red and irritated when I wake up and burn a lot during the day. I had to stop wearing contacts lenses 2 years ago because I had abrasions on my corneas from the dryness."*   *Mary*

If you've ever seen kittens with gunk (such a technical term!) in their eyes that glues their eyelids shut, you know what we can look like some mornings (minus the whiskers, fur and pink ears).

Various eye irritations, as well as visual problems, may also develop in relation to FMS. Blurring of vision is common. We may also go through numerous vision changes. Again, one must be cautious to rule out other problems. But for many people there is a definite connection between the above eye symptoms and FMS.

Sinus problems and infections, as well as allergies, are also major concerns for many FMS sufferers. They certainly have affected me. I had chronic sinus infections due to allergies for many years.

> *"It started last Friday with some sinus congestion and headache. Finally dropped to the chest last night. Blowing, hacking, wheezing, etc. Chest feels like I've got an iron band around it that someone keeps tightening. I know it's just allergies and FMS."*   *Gail*

Here's Heather's story:

"I had no pain with my FMS/CFIDS until I had been sick for 6 years. I only had frequent bouts of "flu" every other month or more that put me in bed for several days. I would run a fever and ache all over, with heavy congestion. I thought these were sinus infections. I did have a strong tendency to get them. Looking back, I know this was the CFIDS part of the disease. I didn't know what was wrong. I was tested for everything. When my body aches started I had figured out I probably had CFIDS/FMS."   *Heather L.*

(CFIDS stands for chronic fatigue immune deficiency syndrome, and is a newer, more accurate term for CFS.)

Considered more on the CFIDS side of the symptom spectrum are sore throat, painful or swollen lymph nodes, and as Heather mentioned, a fever. I have frequent sore throats; however, I have an unusually low body temperature (not unusual for FMS). Seems 98.6 is an elusive number for most of us!

Dizziness, or vertigo, is often present with FMS. There are many causes of dizziness, including medication, hypoglycemia, shallow breathing, inner ear problems, asthma and low blood pressure. These can all be associated with FMS, so it's no wonder we are dizzy! It can be frightening:

"I am experiencing severe dizziness to the point it scares me because I can't focus on anything and I'm very disoriented. I can hardly type this message because I can't find the keys. Dizziness has been one of my top complaints for the past 7 years and now it's gotten worse."   *Rose*

That was a serious concern about a serious problem, but here's a lighter side:

What could you say about a woman in an evening gown who spins around in circles and doesn't get dizzy? She's all dressed up, but no ver-ti-go!

Skin problems we may experience include crawling feelings, itching, various rashes, burning and pimples. A few experience hyper-sensitivity to touch. Hot and cold sensitivities are common.

> *"I can't tolerate very hot water. I feel like I'm being scalded to death in a very warm shower. In fact, when I'm in a flare, I can hardly stand the sensation of water spraying me. I used to work with a catering company and found that touching dish water and dishes that everyone could tolerate almost put me into shock."*   *Valerie*

I, personally, can't stand cold, whether it be cold air or something touching my skin. The feeling goes beyond discomfort, it's just shocking and unbearable.

TMJ stands for temperomandibular joint and may be a part of the FMS equation. This is the joint where the jaw is attached to the skull, just in front of the ear. Problems with this joint can be very painful.

> *"I often have a terribly stiff and achy jaw. Sometimes it's difficult to eat and I just want to swallow some soft foods and get the meal over with. Since I've heard that TMJ is a symptom of fibro, I'm assuming that's what it is with me. It feels like I'm clenching my jaw and can't stop, even though my jaw is open and seems relaxed."*   *Sheryl*

"Lend me your ears" is a phrase we would like to put to "Norms" when our ears are being mischievous and causing us pain or discomfort. They seem to delight in ringing or making other noises at will, though we would much prefer silence. Then there's the pain:

> *"If I am out in a cool breeze, I will get a severe earache in whichever ear the wind is blowing. It goes away after 20 minutes or so indoors. But now I have gotten some earaches indoors too, during a flare. Makes me wonder if the earaches have been a part of the FMS all along. My eardrum also does a little spasm, making a whop-whop-whop sound in my ear, like there is some miniature person in there, playing the drum!"*   *Lynn*

Many FMS'ers experience a wide variety of hypersensitivities. We are not wimps, this can simply be an agonizing part of FMS. We may be sensitive to light, smell, sound, chemicals, or foods, among others. Here are some examples:

> *"Chemical sensitivity was one of my first symptoms, but back then I was totally clueless, never having heard of such a thing. I would completely zone out in the detergent aisle. My husband would have to take my hand and literally lead me out of the store like a small lost child."*   *Nan T.*

> *"I work in a restaurant, and sometimes I feel like running right out the door, just from the noise, music, talking, clanking dishes and silverware. I've always preferred to have my house silent. I can FEEL the TV on in the other room, even if I can't quite hear it."*   *Helene*

> *"It's looking more and more like the weird little kid (and grown up one) I've always been isn't weird at all -- just a "fellow fms'r". . . I have been called the one with the "bloodhound nose!" My sensitivity to smell is so extreme, I*

often can't stay in a clothing store because the dyes smell acrid and burn my nose. And if I do stay, I get a headache."   *Nancy B.*

These, my friends, are some of the FMS monkeys on our backs out to do us harm. We may have to deal with them, but I'm convinced we have it within our power to one day get rid of them. They will hang on and fight ferociously to keep their place, but it keeps me going to believe we can eventually beat them off and put an end to their reign of terror.

Chapter 4
Personal Page   *Date Written* _____

Other than pain, exhaustion, sleep deprivation, brain fog and depression, these are the "monkeys on my back":

Rashes, can't stand loud noises, hate hot weather (or damp).

This one is the worst for me: ~~dizziness~~ brain fog **because:**
~~It hurts too much.~~ I can't think. I can't remember. Feels like Alzheimers.

Second worst is: fatigue **because:** I can't do what I want.

I take these medications for the symptoms I listed above:
Provigil. Haven't taken yet.
Wellbutrin
Not many medications work.
Celebrex

I have these conditions along with FMS:
Sarcoidosis
Hepatitis C
IBS

Dealing with all these symptoms together makes me feel like: dying.

Other thoughts or insights on this chapter:

Playing in Pain

When team athletes are injured, but continue to play the game, we "Ooh" and "Aah" and exclaim, "My, they are brave to play in such pain!" Playing a game in pain may be admirable, but it also has its advantages, such as the injured area is likely to be prominently wrapped, so it draws extra attention to the player. The player is held in high regard for the ability to continue on in spite of injury and when the game ends, "great going" and "way to hang in there" are dispensed along with an admiring pat on the back. All of the above are the result of continuing to do something highly enjoyable despite pain. But the best part is, the injury, while notably painful, will most likely heal in a matter of weeks. Pain with an end in sight is much easier to take than pain that takes up residence in a person's body and refuses to leave.

Pain is the hallmark of FMS. When you have FMS you are playing in pain every day. No one is standing in line to pat *us* on the back or applaud our efforts. We don't have wraps or casts or stitches or bandages. Our pain is invisible. And it doesn't go away. We must go on in spite of it not only in regard to things we enjoy, but also in daily chores and responsibilities we may wish we could forgo, but feel obligated to complete.

Our pain is a little like the devil himself. While we hate him and wish he would just leave us alone, we do have to marvel at his tenacity. He's quite ingenious in getting to us in any and every possible way. This ingenuity draws our attention and hinders us from fully being who we want to be. So it is with our pain.

Except for "charlie horses" in my legs, especially while I was out for track, I had virtually no muscle pain until about seven years ago. Even then, it was only isolated episodes. I remember the first of many identical incidents. I woke up in the morning and every muscle in my body was cramped. I was in so much pain, I could barely get out of bed. Just all of a sudden, there it was. As it was becoming par for the course, I wondered what in the world was going on with my body. Although I was getting older, this had to be something more than the aches and pains one can expect as the years pile up. After it had happened a few more times, I decided our mattress was the culprit, as it always happened before getting up in the morning. So we ditched it for a pricey new one. Problem solved, so I assumed. I was wrong. These episodes not only continued; they became more frequent. When "full blown" FMS hit, muscle pain went from the realm of being an occasional unpleasant morning surprise to becoming my constant companion.

The pain in my arms and legs (except for torturing cramps) is a piece of cake compared to the pain in my neck, shoulders and back. It can be stabbing, throbbing, tight, aching and vicious. It covers the entirety of my shoulders and back of my neck, while running across the edge of my shoulder blades like a train on a track.

My son and daughter are both in sports and sitting on bleachers at their games for over ten minutes begins to feel like someone is beating on my neck, shoulders and back with a spiked mallet. Having something to lean on helps considerably. But by the time the final whistle blows and one game is over, this old gal is in bleacher agony. I have learned I have to limit myself to one game at a time, as I not only pay immediately, but for a day or two afterwards, as well.

I also had pain in my back due to a bulging disk at the low end of my spine. FMS would latch on to this and intensify the pain. Surgery on the disk a few years ago helped the deep-down, sharp pain, but my lower back still aches. FMS pain tends to attack weak areas, especially where there have been surgeries or other injuries.

I used to pride myself on never having headaches. Of course, pride goes before a fall, and now most days I feel like I've fallen head first out of a two story window. My headaches started in my mid-thirties. As is my pattern with other pain, they started out as just a few here and there and gradually increased. But since "full blown FMS" hit, there is always at least a dull ache present. In the back of my head where my spine starts, there is constant pain. Sometimes my whole head joins the party and riotous fun is had by all – all except me.

The pains I have described are common to FMS. Yet, while my pain is intense at times and while I do always have some muscle pain and a headache, my pain doesn't even compare to that of many with FMS. It can be absolutely debilitating.

FMS pain is versatile and can come in many sizes, shapes, styles and intensities. It can be widespread or localized. It can pierce or it can throb. It can squeeze us in its powerful grip and take our breath away. For some, it has wielded the power to take over their lives.

Any pain is unwelcome, but chronic pain is an excruciating, never-ending battle. It gets under our skin emotionally as well as physically. We tire of it. We tire of people saying, "It surely isn't *that* bad." We tire of having to take medication to ease it. We tire of people saying they know just how we feel. We tire of constantly having to deal, deal, deal with it.

Certainly, people with other chronic illnesses also have to address the pain issue. We don't claim a monopoly on its devastation. I believe the one good thing that can come of our pain is a heightened awareness of the pain of others. We are very aware that what you see is not all there is. We empathize with and believe in other people's pain. In turn, we hope others believe in ours.

Our goal is not to gain sympathy from those without pain. We just want to be understood. Our suffering does not afford us the luxury of carrying on our lives in the same manner we used to, or as "Norms" do. We are, however, doing the best we can, and that's what we need others to understand.

Even though our lives are changed, they do continue. We can still laugh, dream, make a difference, work (to varying degrees), create, love, give, and carry on, although we are playing in pain. Pretty impressive, wouldn't you say!

Here's my pat on the back and "way to hang in there" for everyone suffering from chronic pain. I'm cheering you on and hoping an end to your suffering, as well as mine, will soon become a reality.

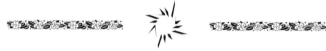

PAIN

Pain is quite invisible
And it's just like the air.
'Cause while you can not see it
There's no doubt that it is there.

Perceptions of pain differ,
In that my headache may feel
Quite different from the one you have.
But both are very real.

You can't diminish someone's pain
By saying, "It's not that bad."
Unless you're there inside their skin,
You can't know the pain they've had.

There's pain that prickles, pokes and prods.
And pain that's underrated.
Pain so intense and piercing
That it screams to be sedated.

If someone tells you they're in pain
They likely mean what they say.
So please don't scoff or laugh or scold.
It could be you someday.

FMS pain is relative
To the pain of the hour before.
There's pain that knocks us off our feet,
Or sneaks in the back door.

We'd rather our pain weren't *relative*,
'Cause relatives stick around.
Better it were a stranger
Who'd pack its bags and leave town.

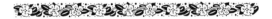

Chapter 5
Personal Page   *Date Written* __⊢9-06__

My daily pain level is:
1   2   3   4   5   6   (7)   8   9   10
Mild   **Moderate**   **Severe**

This (these) is (are) presently my worst pain area(s):
    Back, hands, legs, elbows, shoulders

Other areas of pain are: UTI.

My pain began: Many years ago.

I take this medication for pain: Duragesic Patch 75
                                Vicodin 10

Pain is my worst symptom of FMS   circle one:

            (Yes)   **No**

Pain has changed my life in this (these) way(s):
    I want to die. I cannot enjoy life, my
    babies, my husband.

Other thoughts or insights on this chapter:

Cloak of Exhaustion

This is it for me. This is the symptom that has had the largest impact and caused the most disruption in my life. It's also the one I've tried desperately to talk myself out of. Others have tried, too. I've heard things like, "sometimes it's hard to get going, but once you do, you'll be OK," "if you *act* like someone with energy, you will *become* someone with energy," "if you sleep less, your body will get used to it and you will require less sleep," and my personal favorite, "a more positive attitude will generate more energy." I felt like such a failure when these practical sounding suggestions didn't work for me. I would invariably end up back on the couch and hate myself for being there.

I held such high hopes for Geritol, but for me it proved to be a big disappointment! So did a large variety of vitamin pills (some liquid, allegedly to help absorption) and minerals. I tried many expensive pills and potions, diets, exercise programs, magnets and even cranialsacral therapy. Still the couch beckoned with an actual physical force that I simply couldn't fight. Being diagnosed with FMS helped my state of mind considerably. I had convinced myself I was hopelessly lazy, and it was such a relief to know I was suffering from a fatigue related illness. But it didn't change the reality. I was exhausted. My productive hours in a day were a scant few. Going somewhere for even a couple of hours would wear me out. This is so different

41

from being tired or sleepy. It's a feeling of having all the energy sucked from your veins, then a heavy cloak thrown over you for good measure. A while back I posted the following analogy to my Internet group:

> *I've been following the posts regarding fatigue with special interest, as that is also my worst symptom. I've always thought of it as being covered with a "cloak of exhaustion." This cloak is very heavy and burdensome and I can't get out from under it, no matter how I try. It's always there (with only slight, glorious reprieves), and sometimes it becomes like lead and I simply can't go on. Most of the time, it just makes everything harder. I wish that just for one day, all the people around me could be covered with this cloak, so they would understand the difficulty of living under its weight. I'm looking forward to the day when it will slip off of me and I'll finally be free of its burden. I wish this not only for myself, but for all who are struggling under the cloak. What a great day it will be when we are free of it. (I plan on stomping on mine!)*

I've heard of people in a crisis situation displaying super-human strength by lifting a car off someone crushed beneath it, or performing some other amazing feat. We all know the explanation for this phenomenon is an adrenaline rush, which lasts just long enough to get the critical task completed. I liken this to when I go out in public. I can "pump myself up" and no one will suspect that I'm performing a feat that is out of the ordinary for me. They would never imagine that I collapse from exhaustion the minute I get home. On really bad days, I can't go out at all. On bad days, the "public adrenaline" lasts about an hour. On good days, four hours usually peaks me out. On very rare, really good days, I feel like a normal human being. That's a great feeling, but really brings home the stark contrast between my usual days and what a normal day should feel like. I hate the trip back to my daily reality after one of my rare, great days.

A particularly difficult situation is when I'm at Wal-Mart or the grocery store and exhaustion bears down on me like green on peas. We live 17 miles from town, so even after I've dragged myself through the check-out line, the major challenge still looms ahead. It is absolutely torture keeping myself awake and alert enough to stay on the road going home. Even when I get home, I have to at least unpack the cold groceries. By the time I'm done, I'm about to pass out from the anguish of my exhaustion. It's not often I get stuck in this situation, but when I do, it's like being in a nightmare where the only way to wake is to sleep.

The Bible tells us we are not to covet anything of our neighbors. But I must confess my sin; I covet the energy of the people around me. I am hopelessly jealous of their full, active lives. I despise not being able to be a more energetic mother, wife and friend. I would love to have a clean, neat house and fix awe inspiring meals. I would love to play tennis and walk around museums and spend a day shopping with friends. I would love to be able to work away from home several days a week. But the energy to do those things is just not there. Sometimes I feel like describing myself as a wife, mother and couch accessory!

Although there are times I feel very much alone with this disabling fatigue, I know I am not. Exhaustion is the worst symptom for many with FMS, and the major symptom for those diagnosed with CFS. There are so many of us out there who have limited choices in regard to work, leisure, family and friends, because of extreme exhaustion. Every day is cut short by our energy limitations. Rare days without exhaustion are a priceless blessing to us. We relish every hour that we are able to be active, whether having fun or being productive. Each moment containing a spark of energy is a gift we never want to part with. But like a boomerang, the horrible fatigue always comes back.

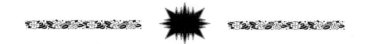

FATIGUE

Fatigue – a nasty little word
Whose meaning I'd rather not know.
Unfortunately we're quite intimate,
As it follows me wherever I go.

My kids ask, "You up for some basketball?"
I sadly reply, "I just can't do it.
Any strength I had has now expired
And I'm stumped as to how to renew it."

A friend approaches me with a plan
That takes more might than I can muster.
I hate to let her down like this.
I've turned into a real fun-buster!

My husband says, "Let's go out tonight,
We'll go to a restaurant and eat."
While this is something I love to do,
I pass, 'cause I'm simply too beat.

Fatigue has locked me in its grip.
It's not about to set me free.
I resent its dogged persistence.
I wish it'd just leave me be.

Time and again I've heard it said,
"Where there's a will there's a way."
If that's the case, this wretched fatigue
Will be gone from me someday.

But for now, it's always here.
Its toll on my life, far-reaching.
Yet for every challenge, a lesson to learn.
I pray I don't miss what it's teaching.

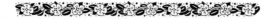

I wonder if fatigue has been my companion for so long, I won't recognize myself when it's gone. How intriguing it will be to see this person emerge from under all the layers of exhaustion. Yes, it will still be me, but it will feel like the *real* me has just been released from prison. I believe personality traits will be exhibited that I've forgotten I ever had. Gee, I hope they are positive ones!

I find great satisfaction in helping other people. Before my fatigue reached this degree of severity, I volunteered in whatever capacity I could. It has been difficult to give up this part of my life, but regrettably I've had to. My family comes first and I feel my limited energy should go to them. Yet even they get pitifully shortchanged. We all have to barter with our time, it's just that extreme fatigue leaves us so much less time to barter with. And the quality of that time often leaves much to be desired. Writing this book is taking more time away from my already diminished days. Our house, long neglected, has now been designated a trash heap – by me anyway. (This is one result of my fatigue the kids couldn't care less about. It doesn't look THAT bad is a frequent comment. I wish it did bother them more, they'd be more apt to help clean!) Frozen pizzas are a hot menu item in our family. Trips to town result mostly from matters of extreme urgency, like no toilet paper (or frozen pizzas). Paper plates and plastic silverware are calling out to me from the grocers' shelves. By the time I get around to calling friends, they have to ask, "Sue who?" (That one's not really true, but you get the point!) However, since I can no longer volunteer, writing this book is fulfilling my need to reach out. The great thing is, I can do it in the comfort of my own home. In other words, I can hit the couch whenever I need to. And I need to a lot.

My #1 health goal is to have more energy. If this is your goal, let's make a pact to persevere until one day we have the life we now only dream of. I personally won't rest until that day comes (figuratively speaking, of course)!

Chapter 6
Personal Page   *Date Written* _____

My level of fatigue is:

1	2	3	4	5	6	7	8	9	10
Mild				Moderate					Severe

My fatigue began:

I've tried these remedies for fatigue:

Fatigue is my # ____ symptom.

Other factors or illnesses that affect my fatigue:

A few things I can't do now, but would love to do when my fatigue lets go of its grip:

An analogy of my fatigue:

Other thoughts or insights on this chapter:

It's So Depressing

Depression. A majority of us were diagnosed with it early on in our search for answers. Maybe it was present within the framework of FMS, maybe not. But the important thing to understand is that our symptoms are not the *result* of depression.

This is our situation: we are faced with a multitude of symptoms, either slow onset or sudden. In the midst of pain, fatigue and muddled thinking, we begin an often anguishing search for answers. This may last years and include a staggering number of tests (some invasive or painful). We may also have to put up with many insults to our character, such as doctors telling us it's all in our heads and others telling us to just get over it. When we are finally diagnosed, many doctors, rather than trying to learn more about FMS and the best methods of treatment, tell us FMS doesn't exist. Our lives as we knew them have come to a halt. We are faced with so much loss. People don't understand us. No one has any easy answers for us. Doctors who DO believe in FMS tell us there is no cure. Seems to me even the most stalwart among us would find these circumstances depressing.

I'm not denying the forceful roll depression plays in FMS. There may well be a physiological component. Since FMS affects every cell, it seems reasonable that it could attack the area of our brains dealing with emotion. However, just as pain didn't cause FMS, neither did depression. They are both simply parts of the whole.

Dr. Kevorkian is well aware of the despair that may accompany FMS. More than one of his "patients" have been FMS sufferers. How tragic it is that he is the one person they felt could "help" them out of their misery. If only they had known there is hope. Maybe they just didn't know how to begin "parting the fog."

I wrote the following poem for a junior college assignment. It was about a friend of mine in the midst of a deep depression.

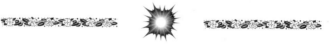

APPEARANCES

People can hide their feelings
If they're feeling low,
But others can usually tell
By the expression their faces show.

Some have learned to be quite clever.
Their faces are a disguise.
They force a smile upon their lips
And wipe the sadness from their eyes.

They go through life pretending.
And no one thinks to ask
If they are feeling any pain.
They hide it with a mask.

Loneliness is covered
By a look of gaiety.
Their faces show contentment,
And that's all that people see.

We must care enough to look closely,
Since outward appearances lie.
Or someone who seems to love life
May decide it's better to die.

Interestingly, I began suffering from depression several years later. My bouts with it have usually been circumstantial and thankfully never to the point of wanting to end my life. I do seem somewhat prone to mild depression. Certainly my trials with FMS haven't helped that tendency. Thankfully, I have reached a point in my life in which I'm currently not suffering from depression at all. Sure, I get discouraged from time to time; we all do in living under the shadow of FMS. I'm also very emotional and there are times I can cry at the drop of a pin (or a touching commercial, sideways glance, or even from losing my glasses one too many times!). However, this is different from the gloomy hopelessness of depression.

Some years ago, when doctors diagnosed me with depression, I don't believe it was what I was actually suffering from. I was just plain tired and in pain (hypothyroidism, FMS combo?). If there was depression, it was mild and due to my circumstances. When I was put on anti-depressants, I gave them sufficient time to help my symptoms. I eventually stopped all of them as they did absolutely nothing for me. I think I tried three different kinds at the insistence of my doctors. This was a simple matter of misdiagnosis. Earlier, when I was suffering from major depression, I didn't get the help I needed. This major depression hit in my twenties. It prompted this poem, which I didn't even bother to title. Unfortunately, some of you in the throws of depression will relate:

Someone help me, take my hand.
Hear me, and try to understand.

I'm dying inside, can't you see
I'm not the person I used to be.

I need someone to guide me through
This loneliness life's led me to.

Into my life people come and go.
They don't really see my misery though.

My eyes look out, but all they see
Is emptiness in front of me.

How much more can I take
Before the pressure makes me break?

Know me, hear me, be my guide.
Please don't let me die inside.

This is miserable stuff to deal with. Many of you know from whence I speak. I know many FMS'ers must take anti-depressants to lift the weighted cloud of despair. For some they work; for some they don't. Some of you may be ready to give up the fight. I implore you to hang on, know you are not alone, and find something in which to hope. Tomorrow can be different. I'm pulling for you and hoping it will be.

Chapter 7
Personal Page   *Date Written* _____

I would rate my depression at the moment (circle one):

Non-existent   Mild   Moderate   Moderately Severe   Severe

My depression started:

These are some of my experiences with depression:

I'm currently on this medication for depression:

It works for me (circle one):
   very well   fairly well   so-so   poorly

My depression feels like:

Other thoughts or insights on this chapter:

Stumbling and Bumbling

Since our bodies and emotions are such a wreck, you'd think FMS would at least leave our minds alone, but no, they take a turn for the worse as well. The "technical" name for this annoyance is brainfog or fibrofog. To put it more formally: our cognitive skills become impaired (which amounts to our brains taking off for spring break, then deciding to stay and take up residence in Cancun!). This is the part of FMS that can leave us embarrassed, exasperated, humiliated, frustrated and searching for the meaning of life, as we already know we can't find anything else. The up side is that this symptom allows us to learn not to take ourselves too seriously (sometimes anyway).

How is one to explain this "altered state" while still under its influence? The word disoriented comes to my otherwise blank mind. It could be said that we are somewhere out in left field, most likely at the wrong ballpark! Yes, we must admit, we do dumb things – often – OK, every day (at least that's been my experience). Trust me, we are not working on our "dumb blond" image; our ding-y behavior is totally out of our control.

I can't speak for others (often I can't even speak for myself) but this symptom irritates me to no end. I have an awful time trying to carry on a conversation. I lose simple words and stare dumbly at the person I'm talking to, in hopes that they can fill in the blank. Also, in mid-sentence I may suddenly lose my train of thought (this train is bound for oblivion!). Sometimes I do make it through a whole sentence, but just as I'm about to breath a sigh of relief, I realize (or it's rudely pointed out to me) that I've used one or more words completely contrary to what I meant to say. I'd be much better off if I just kept my mouth totally shut at all times. However, my troubles wouldn't stop there.

My short-term memory is practically non-existent. I've lost everything I own at least once. I forget how old I am, which can be quite advantageous! I forget the names of people I've known for years and certainly can't remember the names of people I've just met. I have to write these sentences really fast or I forget where I'm going with them. I stand in a room or at an open cupboard or refrigerator and wonder what on earth I'm doing there. I'll be driving the car and not have the slightest idea where I'm going. If I do remember where I'm going, I may forget how to get there! The worst thing I've forgotten was that someone had died. That wouldn't have been so bad, except I asked a relative how he (the deceased) was doing! Another snafu that could have been avoided, had I kept my mouth shut.

Then there are the "spaced out" occurrences. I've poured juice on my kid's cereal, put my purse in the freezer, slammed my head in the car door (ouch!) and wasted time looking for glasses that were right on my nose!

Here's a fibrofog moment I posted to my Internet group:

> *It was cold with light freezing rain when I took my daughter to her orthodontist appointment this morning. As I sat in the waiting room reading, I heard the receptionist suddenly say, "I wouldn't want to be playing soccer today." I looked up and she was looking at me. It seemed a bit odd that she would say that out of the blue, but I always say weird things out of the blue, so I simply replied, "I wouldn't either." (Never mind that I've never played soccer in my life.) She went on, "It's just too nasty to play soccer on a day like this." I quipped, "I would sure think so." She said, "I wouldn't even want to be out watching it on a day like this." I agreed, "Me neither!" She grimaced, "I just don't like the cold weather." I nodded,*

"Oh, I know! I can't stand the cold. I can't even stand going to football games."

At that moment it registered that she had a phone to her ear! She soon hung up and I smiled at her and said, "I just realized you were talking on the phone and not to me!" She said, "Yeah," and although I'm riddled with pain and fatigue today, I burst out laughing. She was amused and forgiving of my social blunder. Luckily, no one else was in the waiting room at the time. I prefer displaying my goofy behavior to one person at a time!

Thankfully (or should I say unfortunately) I'm not alone. I've read and heard many accounts of incidents resulting from the fog of FMS. Among them: using room freshener as deodorant (no biggy, nice fresh smell either way); buying the same book twice within a 1/2 hour period (actually, a smart move, as one will inevitably get lost); wearing mis-matched shoes in public (simply making an FMS fashion statement); struggling to get out of the car with the seat belt still on (at least in that instance one wouldn't fall out of the parked car); in a roomful of people, introducing oneself as the person to the left (could be a Freudian slip, may want to be that person); and swallowing the pet's medicine (it's good to find new ways to interact with our pets!). And this is just the tip of the exasperating fog-covered iceberg!

But, you may say, everyone does dumb things; this is not exclusive to FMS. Very true. Those of us with fibrofog just do them on such an unfailingly consistent basis.

Sometimes there is nothing humorous about the fog. It can be a huge liability in the workplace. Very intelligent people have found themselves in this fog, with their jobs suddenly compromised. Although I don't work outside the home, for me it can be distressing to not comprehend what's going on around me. I often don't understand what people are saying to me. I hate the times I have to read things over and over before they "sink in." Keeping track of kids' school events, lunch money, notes to sign, and clothes to send, is all very difficult for me. I even have trouble following some movies: too many characters to keep track of, the people talk too fast, background music distracts me, the plot is too complex. Thank God for movies like "The Wizard of Oz," which happens to be my all time favorite! Anyway, it's oppressive to feel the world around me is moving along at a normal speed, while my brain is stuck in slow motion.

Then there is the clutz factor. Poor coordination is the Laurel and Hardy symptom of FMS. I'm always tripping over my own feet (as well as those of others). I lose my balance when simply standing and may sway into people (that's a strange sensation). Like a drunk being kicked out of a bar, I may stagger or bump into people and things. I hate to admit it, but it was comforting to learn that others with FMS are often as wobbly as I; without being drunk or high on drugs. Why FMS brings such a lack of coordination to both body and mind is a mystery to me. I do know these two deficits in combination can be lethal.

The following poem is a fictionalized account, but could well be true in the world of stumbling and bumbling we may face as part of FMS:

LOST IT

Someone told me to my face
That I have lost it totally.
"Humph," I said, "Of all the nerve.
How can you think that of me?"

"It's not lost, it's just misplaced.
What is it I was looking for?"
As I looked, in vain (for what?)
I rammed my head into the door.

"That really hurt," I then proclaimed
In slightly different words.
"Now what were we just talking about?
This headache's for the birds."

This person said, "It seems to me
Your thinking has been horrid.
Soon we will be hanging
A 'FOR RENT' sign on your forehead."

"I have seemed somewhat foggy,"
I lamented through the blur.
"It's one of the symptoms of FMS."
This person replied, "Yeah, sure."

"You don't believe me, do you," I sighed,
"But I won't let that get me down."
Then turning with dignity to leave
I promptly tumbled to the ground.

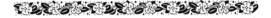

Chapter 8
Personal Page   *Date Written* _____

My fibrofog is (circle one):   no big deal   mildly amusing

an occasional nuisance   a constant annoyance   a royal pain

Fibrofog has affected how I view myself in this way:

Brainfog has affected how I view the world around me in this way:

I'm very aware of brainfog when I try to:

This is my most embarrassing fibrofog moment (that I will admit to):

Here are a few other fibrofog moments:

Other thoughts or insights on this chapter:

Oh, What a Night!

Going to bed should be a time to relax and restore one's body in preparation for the next day. For millions of people this is not the case. FMS sufferers are right there at the head of the class in inability to get a good night's sleep.

It seems like such a simple task to accomplish. Just shut your eyes and float into la-la land. But to us, la-la land may as well be Timbuktu.

There are several different levels of sleep. Getting to the deepest level, which is the one responsible for restorative benefits, is usually an impossible dream for us (pun intended).

Speaking of dreams – aren't they interesting! FMS seems to produce a bumper crop of bizarre dreams and nightmares. I can certainly attest to that. A few years ago I was having incredibly crazy dreams. Everything was fragmented. There was no cohesive thought. These dreams jumped from one scene to a completely unrelated one. Even words did not make sense in relation to each other. (If you are thinking, "So it is with this book," I'm in trouble!) It was unnerving to wake up and consider that something must be really out of whack in my mind for me to dream this way. Although I still have nightmares and strange dreams on occasion, the truly bizarre dreams have thankfully gone away. It's too bad I can't report such improvement of my daytime brain. I'll just need to exercise more patience on that one!

Another weird thing about my dreams is that sometimes I begin to dream even before I'm fully asleep. I know this is true because I feel myself doing it. I realize we are supposed to dream during REM (rapid eye movement) sleep, but occasionally that's not how it works out for me. I've wondered if this is part of the sleep dysfunction of FMS. Then again, my body and brain never do anything in the usual manner, so it could just be me.

Our sleep difficulties fall into the "which came first, the chicken or the egg" category. Are we sore, exhausted, depressed, and have foggy brains because we don't get restorative sleep; or do we not get restorative sleep because we are sore and our bodies and minds are unable to function properly? In either event it's a vicious circle.

While some FMS'ers have difficulty falling asleep, others fall asleep easily but wake frequently throughout the night. Then there are the early wakers who never manage to go back to sleep. The extremely unfortunate are afflicted with a combination of the above.

Most FMS books give hints for getting better sleep. I've been helped by the following: staying away from caffeine (chocolate included) after 2:00 p.m., taking calcium with magnesium right before bed, getting some exercise during the day and not drinking too much water before bed (we all know where that leads). I sleep fairly well now, most nights.

Because FMS bladders often feel full even though they may not be, we may make frequent trips to the bathroom at night. This doesn't help matters much! Neither does restless leg syndrome, which starts when one is trying to fall asleep. It begins as an aching, heavy feeling in the legs and results in the inability to hold them still. Add to the mix leg and foot cramps, a racing mind, itches, twitches, congestion, night terrors, night sweats, pain, pain and more pain, and you have a perfect setup for a disastrous night's sleep. Plus, many of us have snoring partners (I refuse to name names on the grounds that it might incriminate me). My husband, the person whom I didn't name in the preceding sentence, also wakes early and begins to stir just as I am otherwise at the point of getting some good sleep

(I'm a frequent waker). It's enough to make the bedbugs consider a change of location! I bemoan my nighttime miseries in the following poem:

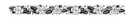

A NIGHT(MARE)

"Oh What a Night" is a great old song,
But I'm feeling so out of tune.
My mind and my body won't give it a rest.
I might as well howl at the moon.

I'm punching my pillow and kicking my legs.
Is this what is known as a punch-kick?
All this commotion while trying to sleep
Is enough to make anyone sick.

So I call in an army to help me,
In the form of little white sheep.
But they thumb their noses and run away.
Reminds me of Little Bo Peep.

Replacement sheep come and I give to them
Encouragement and lavish praise.
But they too fail to make me sleep.
Can't *count* on good help these days!

So, adeptly I solve the world's problems.
And worry 'bout things great and small.
My muscles hurt and my head feels like
It's been forcefully slammed in a wall.

Before the sun begins to rise
My senses are starting to dull.
I finally sleep, but frightfully dream
I'm the next victim of "Hannibal."

I pray for the Lord to rescue me
From the miseries of the night.
He answered long before I asked
When He said, "Let there be light."

Yet morning holds its own set of concerns. That is when stiffness takes center stage, making it an accomplishment of epic proportions to assume an upright position! Also, because of such a frustratingly active night, exhaustion often makes FMS'ers (this one anyway) loath to get up and face the day. Consequently, a tad bit of grumpiness may ensue.

I am thankful for two things: 1. I no longer have babies to get up and feed in the night. I am pretty much left alone to sleep, or not to sleep (except for my dear husband's unwitting contributions to my wakefulness). 2. While my head is on my pillow, I can look out my window and see the stars and watch the lights from planes move off into the distance. This is relaxing and takes the edge off my "must get to sleep" self-talk.

The sleeplessness of FMS is often a symptom which requires medication. Because of the critical role of sleep, my take on this is – do whatever gets you through the night (with at least a few winks). I went the medication route for a few years, but when I had to raise my dose more and more and it seemed to help less and less, I quit. As with other medications, I was no worse off for quitting them and possibly it even helped me. I know this would not be the case for everyone.

The childhood prayer which begins "Now I lay me down to sleep," has become for us a plea rather than a statement. Thus, I end this chapter with a wish that just for tonight, you will sleep deep and dream sweet and greet the new day rested and restored. Contrary to what I said earlier, a good night's sleep is not an impossible dream!

Chapter 9
Personal Page   Date Written _____

I suffer from the following (check those which apply):

_____ **I have trouble falling asleep**
_____ **I wake frequently during the night**
_____ **I wake early and can't go back to sleep**

These factors contribute to my sleeplessness:

I take these medications to help me sleep:

Typically my dreams are:

This is how I feel when it's time to get up:

My quality of sleep is (circle one): Good Fair Poor
What sleep?

Other thoughts or insights on this chapter:

So Much Loss

It's staggering to think of the losses FMS perpetuates. While these unwanted consequences of our disease vary greatly with each person, I think it's safe to say none of us escape the experience of some loss within the framework of FMS.

Following is a sampling of the losses we may face: people with FMS may lose their jobs or a lucrative career due to pain, exhaustion and brain fog, we may lose friends who just don't understand our illness, we may no longer be able to pursue hobbies we once enjoyed and we may need to cut back on exercise, as too much can make FMS worse. Losing the freedom to go about our normal lives is a loss most of us are dealt and to many of us the loss of productive hours in our days is sobering. We suffer the loss of credibility among the human race at large, which is unfair, unfortunate, and undeniable. Finally, it's not uncommon for people with FMS to see a marriage come to an end because the spouse can no longer cope.

One by one these losses impact our lives. They can be even more devastating than the illness itself. We have been thrown into a world completely different from that of a well person, although we may look perfectly fine to others. This is a world where many things are taken away and we have to put up a vicious fight to get them back.

Some have lost nearly everything they held dear due to FMS. I don't know precise statistics on how many have suffered this profoundly, but I do know it's no small few. These people, who have endured so much, were the inspiration for the following poem:

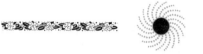

ONE LIFE

This is a story about a girl
Who appeared to have it all.
Quite happily married, a great career,
'Til fibromyalgia came to call.

She didn't know what was happening.
Nothing was working out as it should.
Racked with pain and numbing fatigue,
She struggled on as best she could.

Her world as she had known it
Then slowly came crumbling down.
The career that she had dearly loved
This illness proceeded to drown.

Her mind that was so sharp and clear
Was overtaken with constant fog.
The energy level she'd taken pride in
Sank like a stone in the bog.

All the symptoms of misery
Took too much strength to fight.
"Why was this happening, what could she do?'
She lay awake wond'ring at night.

Then one day her husband said,
"You're not the person you used to be.
You have to take control of your life.
I need you, can't you see."

He tried in vain to understand.
But for him it was just too much.
He left and she reached out desperately
For something on which to clutch.

She did find something to cling to
Right there within her mind.
A single word, yet in her search
Hope was the answer she'd find.

Though never an easy battle,
Hope keeps her going until
Her fight with the monster that is FMS
Will see her go in for the kill.

Other than the major life changing losses, we are vulnerable to a host of other annoying losses as well. And of course, there are the losses that accompany the symptoms: loss of muscle tone, skin quality, sleep, brain clarity, visual acuity, energy, balance and so on.

I have suffered my fair share of losses, yet mine are mild compared to what some people with FMS have experienced. I lost the ability to work full time. I had to give up teaching piano lessons and doing volunteer work. I can no longer be very active with the music in my church. It's difficult to play tennis, bowl or go for long walks. I used to love spending a day shopping with friends, now it would just make me miserable. While I haven't exactly lost friends, some have distanced themselves. To put it more accurately, because of FMS, I have kept more to myself and they haven't made an effort to understand or stay close. I've lost the energy to be the kind of wife and mother I want to be. I've lost my enjoyment of yard work and gardening, it just wears me out too much. I've lost the ability to keep a clean house. Oh, and here's another one of my painful losses:

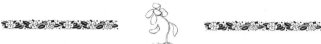

A BITTER LOSS

Have I really been so bad to you
You've felt you have to leave?
Don't you know that when you do
So bitterly I grieve?

We've been together for so long,
Since before I had turned two.
At times you're quite rebellious,
Still, I've come to count on you.

But now you're slowly leaving me
And I am filled with pain
To know that our relationship
Is going down the drain.

I never thought it'd come to this.
It just does not seem fair.
I'm losing such a part of me.
So long, my precious hair!

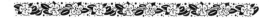

My husband could join me in lamenting this loss as well! But in the scheme of things, this one really isn't that important.

Some of our losses are heart wrenching. If every tear shed due to FMS losses were gathered together, they would, no doubt, fill Lake Michigan. Yet, I believe these losses have the potential to lead us on a new path, give us a fresh perspective and help us to find strength we were unaware we had.

I also believe we should mourn our losses, rather than deluding ourselves by claiming they don't matter. After mourning, we should round the bend and move on in the direction our lives now take us. I hope to meet you on the road to recovery.

Chapter 10
Personal Page   *Date Written* _____

The major losses I've experienced due to FMS are:

These are some of my other losses:

I feel I have suffered [more   average amount of   less] loss than the people around me.

I feel I have suffered [more   average amount of   less] loss than others with FMS.

My losses have affected me as a person in this (these) way(s):

Other thoughts or insights on this chapter:

Hanging In and Holding On

Some days I don't cope very well. When my pain level is high, fatigue relentless, and brain numb, coping isn't even a consideration. My task at hand is simply to come out alive at the end of the day! The single goal I strive for is to not rip apart family members. That goal, too often, is not attained! On these days, my best bet is to stay in bed with the bedroom door shut and emerge only in correlation with hunger pains. (We have a master bathroom, so I don't have to re-enter the world to tend to that business.)

It isn't easy to cope with an illness that is as misunderstood as FMS. We have to cope with debilitating symptoms, disbelieving doctors, unconcerned people and loss. At the same time, we are fighting our own doubts and insecurities. All this we do while attempting to hold on to our wits and some semblance of the person we know we still are inside.

Again, informative books on FMS give many hints on how to cope with chronic illness. As for me, I just try to get through each day as best I can. I try to strike a balance between doing so much I will pay later (some days I physically can do little to nothing) and doing enough to bolster my feelings of self-worth and accomplishment. It's a delicate balance to attain and sometimes I slip off the high wire and land with a thud (usually on my pillow).

I think my best coping strategy has been learning to say "no." In the small-town community I live in this has been difficult. Everyone is expected to contribute to the good of the community. People talk if you say "no" to a request or don't attend this meeting or that social function. While I *want* to do what I can, I'm getting better at recognizing the commitments that would compromise my health and I turn them down. And I've come to the point where it doesn't matter as much to me what people think, although it still does too much. It's hard to realize some people may think less of me because they don't understand the nature of my illness. But when I stop and consider I'm accountable only to God, it makes it easier.

The main coping aid the majority of FMS sufferers rely on is medication. I've whittled mine down to Synthroid, Guaifenesin (my treatment medication), a hormone replacement pill and an occasional pain pill. I also take calcium and am trying to get in the vitamin habit again. I used to take a dizzying amount of medication. I'm so thankful I've been able to back away from it. I know many absolutely *need* one, two or several medications to get severe symptoms under control. Even though they may help, it truly is a pain to have to mess with them. Looking back to my "plethora of pills" days prompted this poem:

PILL TAKING BLUES

I've so many pills in my medicine chest.
This is a part of my life I detest.
Between pink pills and blue pills, large ones and small
It's simply too hard to keep track of them all.

Pills for depression and pills for the pain.
So many pills that it drives me insane.
Pills for my thyroid, for mood swings – hormones.
Tums with its calcium strengthens my bones.

Then there's a pill to help me sleep.
None of these pills, by the way, come cheap.
Without this white pill my sinuses block.
Seems I am pill-taking 'round the clock.

The thing that confuses me most of all
Has to do with my sense of recall.
As I reach for a bottle I promptly forget
Whether or not I've taken these yet.

Some of the pills I take when I get up.
With others the water must be a full cup.
These with my breakfast, these right at noon.
The mid-afternoon ones I'll have to take soon.

Right before bed I've a ritual to keep,
Taking more pills before going to sleep.
I need to watch out because some pills don't mix.
You see, all these pills have me in quite a fix.

I've so many pills, 'cause I've so many ills.
All of this pill-taking gives me the chills.
But as it stands now, I need help through the day.
I pray that it won't always be this way.

I'm sure each of you would love to be able to flush your pills down the stool. However, they offer help, and help is something we sorely (woops – another pun!) need.

The song "One Day at a Time," is one I've sung at several funerals. The chorus begins: "One day at a time, sweet Jesus, is all I'm asking of you. Just give me the strength to do every day what I have to do." This could be our battle cry. For while we need to set goals and dream dreams of a better tomorrow; no matter how difficult, we must live the present day. Thankfully

in life, we are only required to hang in there one day at a time.
Yet, even one day can bring the feeling that all is lost and
there's no use to keep trying. Don't let yourself give in to this
faulty thinking, tempting though it may be. If you feel you have
nothing left and just can't cope any longer, read through this
poem. Maybe it will make hanging in and holding on seem like
a more appealing option.

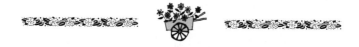

NEVER SAY "ALL IS LOST"

I need the strength to persevere
Though life has dealt me a blow.
I still want to hold my head up high
With courage, so others will know:

No matter how hard a life can be
To never say, "All is Lost."
You simply find courage to carry on
In spite of the pain and cost.

I know it's there within my soul
To live my life graciously,
While fighting this illness with all my might.
I won't simply "let it be."

I hope to win this struggle I'm in.
For there is so much at stake.
I refuse to let FMS ruin my life,
For others, as well as my sake.

May I learn new ways of coping,
So to see my ineptness gone.
And learn to delight in the strength I employ
As I "keep on keeping on."

Daily trials will test my resolve,
But to each day there's always an end.
I will take my lumps and pick myself up,
Then start each day fresh once again.

Chapter 11
Personal Page   Date Written _____

The biggest challenge I have to cope with is this:

I handle that challenge in this way:

These are my FMS coping strategies:

I cope [better   worse] than I did a year ago.

I'm not very good at coping with:

I've learned to cope well with this:

Other thoughts or insights on this chapter:

12

The Ripple Effect

The title of this chapter does not refer to what happens to our thighs as we get older and put on a few extra pounds! Rather, it is about the people in our lives who suffer the ripple effect of our FMS.

We have so much to contend with, it's easy to become self-absorbed. We can fall into the mindset of feeling so over-whelmed with our personal plight, we give little thought to how it affects others. No man is an island and this becomes very apparent when dealing with chronic illness.

We may have family, friends, co-workers, bosses, employees or neighbors who are to some degree subjected to the effects of our FMS. To me it's bad enough that I have to go through the hell of this illness myself, but it just crushes me to think of the people who suffer by association.

Of course, my family bears the brunt of my ripple effect. Our kids are seventeen and thirteen now and I know it's been hard on them. Ever since they were little I've suffered from exhaustion. I was able to play with them, take them places (fairs, amusement parks and so on), cook for them, take care of their basic needs, read to them, etc. Sounds like a typical family, and in most ways it has been, except for my nagging fatigue. I was-n't a barrel of fun to be with, since although I could do these things with the kids, I did them in a state of exhaustion.

Consequently, I had a sluggish demeanor and very little patience. I get cranky when I'm tired, so my family would concur that my FMS has not been a pleasant (or even neutral) experience for anyone. I'll never forget one day years ago when I yelled at my daughter, and my son, who is three years older, comforted her saying, "It's OK, she just gets like that."

It's been difficult raising two kids while being so fatigued. It takes energy to discipline and teach responsibility, and although I've done my best, I feel I've fallen short in those areas. And since the arrival of major FMS, the scenario has become even more grim. I've often been unable to cook meals and sometimes have had to miss events involving the kids. I've spent less time goofing off with them or taking them fishing, or even talking to them. When under the cloak of exhaustion and pain, it is hard to interact with people, even those you love the most. But I must say, I'm very proud of our kids and their accomplishments in spite of having such a lethargic mother.

Although I've never been a high energy person, my husband is now stuck with a very different wife from the one he married. So often he has asked me to go somewhere with him and I've had to turn him down. His meals have been basic and uninspiring for years, although I would love to have the energy to make them more enticing. If you are thinking he should fix his own meals, let me clue you in as to what he does for a living. He has a small trucking business, hauling mostly hay, so he spends a lot of time loading the hay onto trailers. He helps out at the family-run elevator. He is a cattleman. He is in partnership with his family in a large farming operation. Last, but not least, he owns a rock quarry. I can not justify expecting him to fix his own meals on a regular basis or even helping around the house. The short time he is at home, he deserves to relax after working such long hours. We have the old fashioned, traditional setup in our household, but I am no June Cleaver! I know my illness has been a disappointment to him and I am so grateful he has stayed with me. He doesn't talk about it much, but I know it hasn't been easy. I was not surprised when I read that the divorce rate when chronic illness is present in one partner is extremely high. It takes a strong spouse to deal with the damaging effects of FMS. And the kids, well, they really have no choice.

The following poem reflects my thoughts about my family:

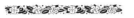 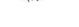

MY FAMILY

My family, you're so precious.
Much more than you could know.
Forgive me for the many times
I've failed to let it show.

I know I'm not the only one
Affected by this illness.
But when there are no words to say
Your love speaks through the stillness.

I've let you down so many ways.
Not been there in your need.
In dwelling on my miseries
Passed up that loving deed.

It's just so hard to carry on
In such fatigue and pain.
I wish some way that you could see
What I just can't explain.

It hurts that I can't be involved
As I would like to be.
Sometimes it seems I've surely failed
In raising my family.

Seems all I have to give you
Is this message I impart:
You always will, each one, possess
A big piece of my heart.

I love you all and always will.
And on the day I'm well
Mere words won't matter near as much,
'Cause then my deeds will tell.

Who has stood by you? It may or may not be family. Family has more of a moral obligation to an ill member, but some will abandon that obligation. Maybe there is someone else who has suffered the ripple effect of your FMS, yet continues to be there for you. Please don't get so caught up in your illness that you fail to recognize their needs. If they have made a significant contribution to your life, be sure they know how much they are appreciated. Being close to someone with FMS is not an easy row to hoe. Show them the following letter, or make up one to give them.

Dear Ones,

You have been put in the position of dealing with an illness that isn't even your own. I'm sorry this burden has been placed on you. I never wanted it to be this way, yet this is our reality. You have handled it better than I ever could have expected or imagined.

Thank you for allowing your strength to be my strength, when I had none of my own. Everyone needs someone to stay by their side, no matter what. You have done that for me. Don't ever think I take your presence for granted. Although I should tell you more often, I am eternally grateful for all you mean to my life.

I am very aware that it hasn't been easy for you to

*accept or cope with my FMS. I know you don't fully under-
stand this illness, but then neither do I. It would have
been so much easier for you to walk away from this hard-
ship. Choosing to stay has proven your strength of character. You passed up the selfish choice out of love and commitment. For that you have earned my deepest admira-
tion and devotion.*

*You have given me so much, while I feel I've been able
to give you so little. I appreciate your generosity of spirit,
which does not ask for an equal return. Maybe someday
I'll be able to repay you in kind.*

*Thank you for believing me when I tell you I'm not
feeling well, although I may look just fine. My credibility
has taken a beating and it means so much that you not
only believe me, but also believe in me.*

*You keep a glimmer of light shining, even in my dark-
est times. I don't know how I could have endured this trial
without your presence in my life. My heart rests assured
that you won't abandon me, no matter how rough it may
get. I feel this assurance because it has been rough, and
still you have stayed.*

*May God richly bless you for your strength, dedication
and love.*

With heartfelt gratitude,

Chapter 12
Personal Page   Date Written _____

The ripple effect of my FMS has been (circle one):

phenomenal   relatively widespread

          moderate   affecting only a few

These are the main people my FMS has affected:

They have been affected in these ways:

Others affected to a lesser degree are:

They have been affected in these ways:

I would like to tell the people who have been affected, yet supportive this:

I would like to tell the people who have been affected and nonsupportive this:

Other thoughts or insights on this chapter:

Varied Reactions

It would be an interesting psychological study to collect data on people's reactions to chronic illness, especially an illness as misunderstood as FMS.

We've had to face the fact that, in general, we don't get the support or sympathy we deserve. We may think it unfair (and of course, it is) but for me this prompted some deep thinking. Let's say I was not familiar with FMS (or worse, misinformed) and I knew someone who looked perfectly healthy. This person was always complaining about this or that pain and was always making excuses not to do something because she was "just too tired." She abandoned commitments and kept more to herself. She claimed this was all due to an elusive ailment called FMS. So I asked my doctor about FMS and he said there wasn't any such illness. In all honesty, this would be my reaction: I would think, "No wonder she doesn't look sick, she really isn't. She must just be lazy, or a hypochondriac. She seems to want everyone to feel sorry for her. Maybe I'll give her the benefit of the doubt and concede she is depressed." It was difficult for me to come to grips with this reaction. The truth is, if I were not experiencing the devastating symptoms of FMS for myself, I probably wouldn't be very tolerant or understanding of an FMS sufferer either. I would try to be, but doubt I would succeed. A tough truth, but I believe it's important to be realistic regarding other people's reactions. Indeed, when in the same position, we may react the very same way others do, although in *our* position, it seems so wrong.

A definitive illness illicits a much different response from one as controversial and misunderstood as FMS. Paula, from my Internet group, explained the difference well:

> *"One of the things that I noticed when I dealt with breast cancer two years ago was how differently I was treated – by everyone! Say the word fibromyalgia and you get blank stares or doubtful looks. . . say cancer and everybody trips over themselves trying to help. I got cards, letters, flowers and meals, and some recognition for the pain and agony I was going through. I said many times during those months, "I sure wish people took the time to understand FMS the way they do cancer." Truthfully, although the cancer surgery and chemo were very hard, I also think dealing with FMS is sometimes just as difficult, especially emotionally. Perhaps it's because there are specific treatments for cancer, a regimen to follow. There is a cell they can see under the microscope. It's just that I get so weary of trying to explain why I can't do things. It's not because I don't want to, it's because I know what it will cost me in pain and sleeplessness, etc."*

There's a cruel irony at play (probably more than one) in FMS. It goes something like this: Our brains are floating around in a muddled fog. Our muscles aren't happy in our bodies, so they tighten up in rebellion and delight in making us sore. Pain screams at us from all directions, striking randomly and mercilessly. Our heads feel like lead balloons dropped on concrete. We could swear someone has sucked all the energy-giving blood from our veins. Our bowels and bladders are in a constant state of confusion. We may be struggling under a cloud of depression. And we look so doggone good!

I suppose we should be thankful people are always telling us how well we look. In reflection, if I had my druthers, I'd rather look good than look like I feel, but it's a deceptive picture. FMS is like the wolf dressed up as Little Red Riding Hood's Grandma. He certainly looked like a sweet little old lady (of course, the snout should have been a dead giveaway) but what was underneath was the truth of the matter. Our outward appearance gives the impression that we are well and adds to the misconception of FMS. My last word on this subject: Go ahead and tell us we look good (only if we really do, of course), just don't assume that means we must be feeling fine, because chances are we aren't.

One mistake I feel "Norms" make is to compare FMS'ers with each other. Even those with mild FMS may compare other sufferers to themselves. For example, if either a "Norm" knows someone with FMS who works full time, or an FMS'er works full time, both may assume everyone with FMS could work full time if they really wanted to. But our bodies react so differently with this illness. Some have a mild case, others a very severe case, while most fall somewhere in-between. The truth is, most of us do as much as we are capable of, at the level we are at.

I believe most people mean well and want to "get it right" in interacting with FMS friends and family members. Here are some good-natured hints for those people:

Realize we have our limits and don't even ask us:

To walk a straight line. Because we tend to be stumbly, the only straight line we can consistently manage is a quick one to the bathroom when irritable bowel syndrome comes to call.

To keep a clean house. We've had to concede that the world won't end because there are dirty dishes in the sink and laundry on the floor. So feel free to clean it yourself... or accept a messy house.

To attend a day long event. Depending on our level of pain/fatigue, our bodies will be crying out "TAKE ME HOME" long before twilight hits.

To snap out of it. Sometimes we are about to snap all right, but the "out of it" part is impossible.

To answer the question "How are you?" with "I'm fine." Gosh, we hate to lie.

To explain FMS in 10 words or less. If you aren't really interested, don't ask, 'cause it may take awhile. If you just don't have the patience, here's a brief synopsis: I'm exhausted, I ache, foggy brain, lots of pain (only nine words!).

To commit to advanced plans. We're still waiting on that shipment of crystal balls to let us know when we'll feel decent enough to go out.

To be cheerful in the mornings. We'd love to oblige, but a myriad of a.m. symptoms prevents this from becoming a reality.

To sit on the floor for any length of time. It could take us days to get up!

To remember what you said two minutes earlier. Fog can descend on the FMS brain and it's gone without warning (what you said earlier, not the FMS brain).

Here are some questions we DO want you to ask, often:

Can I help? The three most beautiful words in the English language (contrary to what you may have heard).

Can you explain? If we stay in bed all day, don't assume we abhor human contact. Ask if it was pain, fatigue, or some other symptom that kept us in bed.

How do you feel about that? It's nice to have someone who will listen to how we feel about the problems FMS creates. So sit down with us and open your ears.

Can I help you find your keys/purse/glasses/mind? Keeping track of things eludes us.

What's your plan to get well? If we have one, we'd love to share it. If we don't, prompt us to find one. Key word: prompt. Don't threaten.

Am I supportive enough? Oh, how we'd love to hear that.

Could I take you out for dinner or fix you something myself? At times, the joy of cooking becomes the chore of cooking.

Do you know how much I care? Enough said.

This chapter wouldn't be complete without mentioning those special friends who do make a continued effort to understand and stay close to us. They work hard at "getting it right" and for the most part, they do.

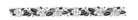 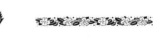

FRIEND

Thank you for being my friend,
Though I'm really not very much fun.
People like people with energy
And alas, it seems I have none.

I want you to know it means so much
That you have stuck with me through all
The canceled plans and constant complaints.
And you never hang up when I call!

Fair weather friends – who needs 'em,
When I have someone like you
Who stays with me 'cause you realize
"In sickness and health" goes for friendship, too.

You deserve one heck of a hug
For being so kind and devout,
And my heartfelt thanks for showing me
What the great gift of friendship's about.

Chapter 13
Personal Page   Date Written _____

The majority of people I've told about my FMS have been (circle one):

Uninterested   Somewhat interested   Very interested

If I were a "Norm" and knew nothing about FMS, I would probably react to someone suffering from it in this way:

If someone tells me I look good, I reply:

My list for "Don't even ask":

My list for "Do ask"

Other thoughts or insights on this chapter:

The Faith Factor

I am a Christian and my faith has been my saving grace, both literally and figuratively. It is such a comfort to know that even if nobody else on this earth understands exactly how I feel, God does. He knows every aspect of me, including my FMS.

When hit with an illness or tragedy, it is natural to ask "why." I did. I even wondered if FMS was punishment from God, although I didn't have a clear idea what for. Of course, I came to realize suffering is simply part of the human condition. We are all going to face suffering because we live in an imperfect world. I wrote the following poem explaining this further:

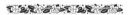

THE ROBBER

A robber of life burst through my door.
In a moment its hostage I became.
Fear gripped me, as I knew if it stayed
My life would never be the same.

While this robber did not kill me,
There's so much it took away.
The burden I was left with
Brought a struggle to each day.

"Why me?" I cried. "What have I done
for my life to turn out so?
I surely don't deserve this fate."
But the robber wouldn't go.

As time went on, I came to see
A truth that helped me understand:
In struggle, I am not alone,
Few lives proceed as they are planned.

To some degree we all are robbed
Of the lives that we desire.
Somewhere, sometime, as we journey on
We'll all walk through the fire.

Whether illness affecting our body or mind,
Or sorrow affecting our heart,
There's one thing the robber of life can't touch.
It has no control of this part.

The soul we possess as a gift from God
Is ours for eternity.
It gives us hope and strength and peace,
Whatever our circumstance be.

When the robber comes, I pray we will not
Let bitterness take control.
But make the choice to find our strength
In the depths of our God-given soul.

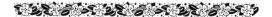

Even when God seems distant, He isn't. My faith is based on the biblical account of salvation, plus my own personal experiences with God's love and grace. I know He is always close to me, even when I can't feel His presence. I have no doubt that God cares deeply about each one of us and if we trust Him, He will see us through each trial we face. You may question why suffering is part of the human condition if God truly loves us. I can't answer that. I do know Christ suffered on the cross not only for our sins, but also to show us He understands our suffering. The why of it, I'm content, will become clear when we get to heaven. In the meantime, my faith brings me peace and comfort in the midst of suffering. God is overseeing the entire picture, while I only see a small part. I'm thankful to rest in the knowledge that He knows best and my life is in His hands.

I write Christian songs and before FMS hit full force, I had a music ministry. I went around to churches and sang my songs. I even made a couple of tapes. At one point I wrote a song for a couple of friends of mine who were going through hard times. Here are two lines from that song:

When it all falls in around us and darkness is all we see
He says, "I am the light of the world, look to me."

It did all fall in around me when FMS launched its vicious attack, consequently those two lines became the essence of my faith. How do people get through suffering without believing in a great and loving God? We are assured of His presence and an end to all our trials in eternity. Without faith as my anchor, I would have a very hard time enduring suffering. Relying solely on myself or other fallible humans would seem to me a risky, lonely course to travel. I'd like to qualify that statement: I do believe God expects me to do all I can and accept help from those He puts on my path, while at the same time relying on Him. This is a much more productive course than passively waiting for Him to act on my behalf. If I do my part, He will more than do His.

I am so thankful for all the factors in my life that have worked together in prompting me to put my trust in God. It has made my burden much easier to bear. May faith lighten your burden, as well. Following is a prayer poem I wrote... feel free to make it your prayer also.

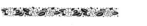

A SUFFERER'S PRAYER

Dear Lord, I am grateful you know me so well
And see in my heart what words can not tell.
While others can't sense what I'm going through,
You know every wish, every fear and pain, too.

Lord, may I not dwell on my own misery.
But reach out to others, then help me to see
I'm not just empowering my fellow man,
But helping myself, as I follow your plan.

Through all of the pain and exhaustion I've known
Help me to sense the great care you have shown.
May I not miss all the blessings you bring,
But seek them, enjoy them and let my heart sing.

Please hold me tight in the palm of your hand.
Give me a heart to understand
That you will stay with me and love me always,
Seeing me through for the rest of my days.

Help me hold my complaints to a minimum, Lord,
Knowing my life in your memory is stored.
Forgive me for blaming you when it's too much,
Rather may I rely on your comforting touch.

Father, I ask that you show me the way
That leads to my healing and a brighter day.
Help me trust in your guidance and rest in your care,
Keeping my hope alive while I'm on the way there.

Chapter 14
Personal Page   *Date Written* _____

My faith is (circle one):   **a critical component in my life**

important to me   something I think about now and then

not very strong   non-existent

I feel faith does (could) help me in these ways:

This is my faith statement:

This is one way God has worked in my life:

Other thoughts or insights on this chapter:

One of the Guais

It is critical to have a plan. FMS is not going anywhere if we don't come up with a way to get rid of it. No plan – no hope of recovery. Most of us have tried a large variety of treatments that have drained our pockets and left us disappointed. We are a bit gun shy when it comes to "helps" or "cures." In our experience, there is very little that has any actual lasting effect on FMS. I know what I'm talking about. I've tried it all (or so it seems). Discouraging? You bet. Still, I refused to give up. I did, however, learn to treat anything that seemed like the genuine article as suspect.

My search for help eventually lead me to the Guaifenesin (pronounced gwī fĕn ĕ sŭn) treatment, pioneered by Dr. Paul St. Amand. One of the reasons I decided to lay aside my skepticism and try this treatment is because it doesn't cost an arm and a leg, and nobody is getting rich by my trying it. As I learned more about this treatment, I came to believe this is the one that will give me back my life. The Internet group I've been quoting from and referring to is the Guai Group. These people have intriguing and encouraging stories to tell of recovery from symptoms. They too had tried it all, and the proof is in the pudding – for a large number of people following this protocol, it works. Here's a shortened version of one of many favorable testimonies to this treatment:

"I guess it is time for an "oldie" to jump in and let you know how GOOD I feel. I have been on Guai for 2 years 3 months (1800mg, no HG diet) and the first 2 years were confusing. But I KNEW that I was not on the same path as I had been – with gradually getting worse each year as I marked birthdays. However, I have just experienced 3 really GOOD months of feeling about 80-90% of what a normal 50 year old would feel.

I know that this would not have just happened on its own, as I was gradually and predictably getting worse for 13 years. I researched this disease and knew a lot and tried many other things, and yet the disease marched on. I could not have heartily recommended Guai in the first 2 years, it was up and down, yet I knew the progress of expected symptoms was altered.

The best advice I can give is to follow the protocol, take the Guai like a vitamin, watch the sals (salicylates) and progress will eventually follow. It is so nice to have a life back again. The verdict is in, Guai works when the protocol is followed."

Barbara

I will attempt to give a very brief explanation of Dr. St. Amand's theory. If you want to learn more and start the protocol, it's imperative you read his book, "What Your Doctor May Not Tell You About Fibromyalgia." Follow this up by getting on the Guai-Support Group web site at netromall.com/guai-support/, and learning everything you can. You really have to be determined to get better, because this is not a quick or easy fix, and you have to follow the protocol exactly for it to work.

Dr. St. Amand doesn't claim to "cure" FMS, but unlike other treatments, Guai goes after the cause of FMS symptoms, rather than covering over them. In a nutshell, Dr. St. Amand theorizes that FMS'ers kidneys don't get rid of phosphates as they should, so they become backed up and accumulate in tissues, muscles and eventually joints. This depletes the energy our cells need, resulting in FMS symptoms. Enter Guaifenesin, which flushes out these waste phosphates, slowly, painfully, but surely. But there's a catch: salicylates (chemical compounds produced by plants, or also made synthetically) take up the same cell receptors as Guai and render it useless. So we must avoid them like the plague. Also, we have to find our correct dosage of Guai, which is genetically determined and different for everyone. Guaifenesin treatment doesn't require giving up present treatments which may be garnering some benefit, with the exception of those employing salicylates. Dr. St. Amand does, however, recommend following the Guai protocol exclusive of other expensive, questionable treatments.

Flushing out the phosphates brings on an exasperation of symptoms and prompts cycles of bad days interspersed with good days. Some (including me) don't have definite cycles, so a reliable way of noting improvement is to get the lumps and bumps on our muscles (extra phosphates) mapped every few months. Mapping consists of a trained person finding them with their fingertips, then marking them on a body outline. Daily journaling of symptoms and feelings is also recommended. There's no doubt it takes hard work and commitment (plus another thing to have to try and explain!), but I'm just glad there's something I can do to help myself.

Before finding my correct dose, I was a bit overwhelmed and confused by the protocol, so I wrote this poem:

GUAI WORLD

Here inside my Guai world
Confusion reigns supreme.
Am I blocking, cycling, at my dose?
Are these things what they seem?

I've been on Guai so long now,
Am I better, worse, the same?
Will I ever be a winner
Of this complicated game?

Those who've gone before me
Say, "Hang in there and you'll see,
This treatment is the answer
If you simply let it be."

Yet that involves so many things:
Patience, determination,
Mapping, dosing, journaling,
The salicylate equation.
(Not to mention the promise of
symptom exacerbation.)

I want so badly to be well,
That I'll walk through this fire.
To come out refined, leave the fibro behind
Is my vision and my desire.

Many others taking Guai related to the sentiments in this poem. In spite of the initial difficulty, we are not about to give up on this protocol, because there are too many success stories. We Guai Group members are extremely resistant to FMS ruining our lives. Guaifenesin treatment as outlined by Dr. St. Amand seems to be my best hope for recovery. Judging from what I know and have heard from others who follow the protocol precisely, I won't be disappointed. Even in the unlikely event that I should be, I'll never give up my quest for wellness.

ONE OF THE GUAIS

After years living in the shadows
With brainlessness, pain and fatigue,
I felt myself destined to live out my life
In the ranks of the sickly league.

Then one of the Guais approached me,
Said, "Our group knows just what you need."
Gave me a book, said, "It will be tough,
But hang in there and you will succeed."

Well, the book talks of pain and a waiting game,
But I soon came to realize
That even though it will mean sacrifice,
I want to be one of the Guais.

Now, these Guais are tough, let there be no doubt.
They know what they want and they go for it.
Courage is needed to join them.
And a will to endure 'til the good times hit.

But for now, others' interest in my decline
Has made for intriguing replies.
For when someone asks me what's happened,
I say I've joined up with the Guais!

Seems they've never quite understood me.
Found me several bricks shy of a load.
But now when I tell them I'm one of the Guais,
They think ALL my bricks fell on the road!

But one of these days it's all going to change.
I'll feel great from my head to my toes.
Oh, what a contrast from where I have been,
Something only another Guai knows.

People will ask how I've come so far,
And my answer will be a surprise:
"I'm proud to say that it's all because
I chose to be one of the Guais."

I'm not telling you this is something YOU should do. It's a very personal decision. I do, however, implore you to look into all the available FMS treatments, then decide for yourself which route you will take. Don't just sit back and let FMS take over without putting up a fight. There is no nobility in remaining miserable and having a negative effect on those around you. FMS will only get worse until a decision is made to do something about it that improves symptoms and gives you hope.

Gentlemen (and ladies) start your engines (if you haven't already) – and let's all leave FMS in our dust!

Chapter 15
Personal Page   *Date Written* _____

This is my plan to get well:

These treatments I've tried for FMS have done little or nothing to help me:

These treatments have had some effect and I want to continue them:

My hopes for recovery are (circle one):   **no hope at all**

slim   **moderate**   **pretty high**

I am definitely going to conquer FMS   **I'm already well!**

Other thoughts or insights on this chapter:

The Power
of Perspective

Keeping things in perspective is an exercise critical to ridding oneself of all that unwanted self-pity. It seems FMS encourages self-pity by virtue of its very nature. The weighted feeling of exhaustion and depression, along with pain, loss, and being misunderstood, gives us ample reason to feel sorry for ourselves. There are two important ways to keep it in perspective: first, look around; second, consider all your blessings.

Suppose there were a gathering in which everyone's burdens were laid out in front of them. If we could leave ours and pick up someone else's, would we? There may be some that appear to be a lighter load than what we bear. Others have laid in front of them incurable cancer or some other fatal illness, abject poverty, a missing child, oppression, tragic loss of family members, confinement in a mental institution, homelessness, wrongful conviction and prison sentence, being victimized by violent crime, and the list goes on and on. There is no way I would willingly trade any of these burdens with my own.

Even within the framework of FMS, I consider myself one of the lucky ones. There are sufferers out there who are the sole income providers for their families, or for themselves. They face enormous pressure on behalf of their families' (or their own) welfare. They feel compelled to work through the pain and exhaustion until they are literally forced to acquiesce to the

105

devastation of FMS. Single parents not only feel this pressure to keep working, they must go home and work just as hard providing quality care for their children. Many end up unable to work and needing disability. From what I understand, fighting to collect it can be an exhausting battle in itself. Whether or not children are involved, a spouse who leaves a marriage because he or she can't cope with chronic illness is always a devastating situation. Some have had to give up careers they attained through years of higher education and hard work. Some have had to give up children to relatives because of an inability to care for them. Yes, I am one of the lucky ones.

Choice is an interesting topic in relation to FMS. In my opinion, we always have some choices. However, the debilitating nature of FMS can and does have a major effect in matters of choice. We can choose to be tough and work through FMS miseries up to a point, but if that certain point is reached, the choice is taken away. The general consensus is that pain allows for more choice than exhaustion. When crushing fatigue takes over, there is not an option to get tough and work through it. When severe enough, it stops you in your tracks. Still there are choices. You may choose to seek out help with any energy you may have. You may choose to see yourself as a survivor and not a helpless victim. That's a choice nobody can take away.

As I've mentioned, FMS is an old illness, although the terminology has changed over the years. In thinking about choice, I considered the plight of slaves with FMS. Most of us have the choice to take care of ourselves, at least to a degree. They had absolutely no such choice. They were forced to perform backbreaking labor that wore down even the healthiest among them. With no visible or detectable illness, their pleas of pain and exhaustion were likely met with a whip. How could they have survived! Maybe they didn't. It is possible that in some cases FMS did kill – either through beatings for not working hard enough, or a body and spirit that simply couldn't go on. It's easy to conceive of a point in which enduring the torturing symptoms under the umbrella of slavery was no longer possible. It breaks my heart to think of the gallant struggles of these people. In light of the forms of oppression and slavery still going on today, everyone reading this should be very thankful not to be suffering from FMS while living under these horrid conditions. Actually, we should be thankful whether or not we have FMS.

Which brings me to the second exercise in waylaying self-pity: be thankful for what you have. We have all been blessed. Some just have to search harder to find their blessings. If you are reading this, here are a few: you have your eyesight; you are able to read and comprehend; you have a few moments to sit and relax; you have many beautiful things to enjoy from nature (one of my favorites is the nighttime sky); there is a God who loves you (whether or not you believe it) and you have food to eat and a bed to sleep in (OK, lie awake in!). You take it from here. I'm sure you can think of many more.

After I had tried many things and before I learned of the Guai treatment, I had a spark of hope, but nothing I knew to try that I felt might be successful. The following poem was written during this period of my life:

THE SMALL THINGS

There are dreams we've had to just let die.
It does no good to question why.
There's still so much we have to give.
We still can dream, we still can live.

Our dreams we've just cut down to size.
Through smaller things we find our thrill.
Our lives take on new meaning.
They are different, but can still fulfill.

Even more we can appreciate
The little things that we hold dear.
Precious things big dreams can't touch;
A smile, a prayer, a loved one near.

Our lives may never be the same,
Yet, we'll grieve who we were and move on.
Then attend to the small things with love and grace,
And our blessings will never be gone.

If through a miracle we are cured,
And our old selves emerge once again,
May the joy we found in small things
Stay with us, even then.

I would like to rescind part of the message of this poem: I don't believe we have to let any of our dreams die. We should always keep the hope our dreams are based on alive. But if our present is restricted to the small things, so be it. Experiencing the joy they bring is an important part of keeping a healthy perspective.

I hope you believe, as I do, that good can be found in even the most dismal circumstances. (I also believe God can help us use our suffering for good if we are open to His leading, but that's another story.) One bit of good that's come from my experiences with FMS is meeting friends I never would have known otherwise. These FMS friends are people I can relate to and share with. While I wish we didn't have the common bond of FMS to bring us together, I am glad for their understanding and friendship. I wrote the following poem before beginning the Guai treatment. While Guai is no magic wand, it just may be the eventual end to my FMS complaints.

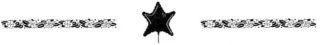

THE MAGIC WAND

Could I wave a magic wand today
And my fibromyalgia would go away,
What aspect would the most joy bring
Were I to ditch this loathsome thing?

To go all day and not need rest
Would surely be the very best.
To know a life with energy
Would be a dream come true for me.

Appealing, too, is an end to pain.
That loss would truly be my gain.
Its lonely invasion can't be seen,
But it's awfully persistent and downright mean.

Having a brain that could think and recall
Would bring the most relief of all.
I stumble and stammer and lose my own name.
Playing the dummy is not a fun game.

Spending each night in a restful sleep
Is a lifestyle change I'd gladly keep.
To waken refreshed with the morning sun
Would surely be half the battle won.

What I *would* miss are the friends I've made.
They've felt this pain, they've been afraid.
In knowing what I'm going through,
They're the ones who have a clue.

A silver lining can always be found
If one makes the effort to look around.
And when I look, what do I see?
These friends who know how it is with me.

I still wish a magic wand would wave,
My life from FMS to save.
Not just for me would I love this done,
But for those in it with me, every one.

I very much want us all to be saved from the miseries of FMS. While we wait, let's consider our blessings, the good that may have come from our FMS and the importance of keeping it all in perspective.

Chapter 16
Personal Page　　　　　　　Date Written _____

This is my current situation (i.e. single parent, no job, etc.):

I consider my burdens (circle one):

easier than most　　　**moderate**　　　**harder than most**

These things are not currently choices for me:

These are just a few of my blessings:

After an in-depth search, I've found this good came from my JMS:

Other thoughts or insights on this chapter:

Letting Hope Reign

I hope this book has fulfilled the intended purpose of putting words to some of your FMS experiences, as well as giving others a better understanding of FMS. My ultimate hope is that it will eventually become a memory book for each one of us. A book that gives us a chance to look back at our struggles and realize how far we've come.

Hope has been a prevailing theme throughout this book. So even if you gain nothing else from reading it, may the hope I've spoken of jump off these pages and into your heart. It surely may be the most critical component to our well-being. It's true that what we hope for doesn't always come to fruition, but that is not ample reason to abandon the feeling of hope. Each day, each situation, brings a new chance for hope. Past experiences shouldn't diminish its power. In fact, its very essence is in looking ahead with confidence, not back with disappointment.

Hope is a little like baking soda, in that it's good for so many things! It draws our attention to the parting of the fog and away from the fog itself. It gives us strength to carry on and refreshes our weary spirits. It brings motivation to act, and last, but not least, it lightens our burden. It is well worth keeping alive.

FMS leaves plenty of room for hope. Researchers and many doctors long for a better understanding of this complicated illness and they will press on until they get it. Even current treatments (in my case Guai) have the potential to free us from symptoms. It's a hopeful time for FMS sufferers. Five or ten years from now will be even better. Just hang on with all you've got to your hope and faith and they will see you through.

HOPE

Hope is the seed planted in our hearts
That must be watered again and again.
For if it dies, we join the ranks
Of sad and desperate men.

Hope keeps us from giving up.
It bolsters our mind and soul.
In matters of the heart, it seems
Hope plays a critical role.

Without it, what is left for us
But to live out the present day,
Not considering that tomorrow
May be better in some small way.

This is a gift God has given us,
More precious than gemstone or flower.
For hope gives direction to our days,
Bringing light to our darkest hour.

If the present is filled with pain and loss,
Hope will bring strength to our life,
And carry us high above the storm,
To give vision beyond our strife.

Yes, hope is the seed planted in our hearts,
To be nurtured with love and care.
It lifts our sights beyond today
So the burdens of life, we may bear.

I leave you to ponder the following Bible verses. May they inspire you to be patient and steadfast in your hope. Just remember, regarding FMS, patience is virtuous, but resignation is disastrous. May hope move you in the direction of a better future. I'm behind you all the way.

Keeping hope before you – journey on!

But hope that is seen is no hope at all. Who hopes for what he already has? But if we hope for what we do not yet have, we wait for it patiently.
Romans 8: 24,25

Be joyful in hope, patient in affliction, faithful in prayer.
Romans 12:12

Chapter 17
Personal Page   Date Written _____

This is what hope means to me:

My biggest hope is:

I plan to keep my hope alive by:

Other thoughts or insights on this chapter:

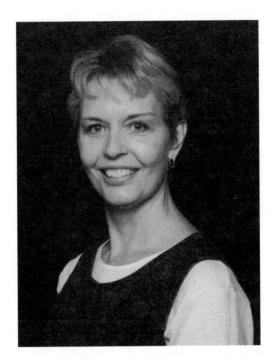

Sue Jones is a wife and mother of two, living in the "Land of Ahs" (Kansas). She was officially diagnosed with FMS in 1997. Her poems relating to FMS have touched the hearts of many with this illness. This is her first book.

Order Form
Parting the Fog

TOTAL

1 book . . . .$12.95 _____

2-3 books . . . .$11.70 each _____

4-5 books . . . .$10.40 each _____

over 5 books . . . . $9.10 each _____

add $3.00 shipping and handling for one book _____

add $.50 S&H for each additional book _____

TOTAL _____

Kansans add 5.4% sales tax _____

TOTAL ENCLOSED _____

U.S. Payment method: ☐ check or money order
☐ Mastercard ☐ Visa ☐ Discover

Card # _____ Exp. _____

Signature _____

Name:

Address:

Phone:

Send Payment to: LaMont Publishing
P.O. Box 125A
Reading, KS 66868

You may also send credit card info by fax: 1-620-699-3819, or call:
1-800-875-2320 between 8:30AM and 7:30PM, Central Standard Time,
Monday - Saturday. All information is secure.

Orders outside the US:
Send International Money Order in US dollars only

of books . . . . _____

Total amount of books . . . . _____
(from price list above)

Canadians add $4.50 S&H . . . . . . _____
plus $.50 for each additional book _____

Other countries: e-mail lamontpbl@osprey.net
for shipping rates to your country.

Add your country's rate . . . . _____

TOTAL _____

Please check if you found this book from the Guai Group website or list ☐